Homeopathic
Color & Sound
Remedies

HOMEOPATHIC
Color & Sound
REMEDIES

REVISED

Ambika Wauters
Dip Hom Med, SHM (UK)

CROSSING PRESS
Berkeley | Toronto

Crossing Press
an imprint of Ten Speed Press
PO Box 7123 • Berkeley, California 94707
www.tenspeed.com

Distributed in Australia by Simon and Schuster Australia, in Canada by Ten Speed Press Canada,
in New Zealand by Southern Publishers Group, in South Africa by Real Books, and in the United
Kingdom and Europe by Publishers Group UK.

Cover and text design by Katy Brown

Library of Congress Cataloging-in-Publication Data
Wauters, Ambika.
Homeopathic color and sound remedies / Ambika Wauters. — Rev.
    p. cm.
  Summary: "Provides guidance on how to use specific homeopathic color and sound remedies
for energy healing; updates to this edition include the addition of sound remedies, new findings
about color healing, and a comprehensive energy assessment guide to help with patient diagnosis"
—Provided by publisher.
  Includes index.
  ISBN 978-1-58091-183-2
  1. Color—Therapeutic use. 2. Sound—Therapeutic use. 3. Chakras.
  4. Healing—Miscellanea. 5. Homeopathy—Materia medica and therapeutics.
  I. Title.
  RZ414.6.W38 2007
  615.8'312—dc22   2007025995

Printed in the United States of America
First printing, 2007

1 2 3 4 5 6 7 8 9 10 — 11 10 09 08 07

CONTENTS

Acknowledgments

I received considerable help in doing the provings, and I would like to say a special thanks to Roger Savage, RS Hom, and Liz Kinsey, RS Hom, both colleagues of Jan Scholten and long-standing homeopaths in Britain. Roger was very supportive throughout my ten years of proving in the UK from 1990 to 1998 and encouraged me throughout. He asked me to speak about my findings at the Society of Homeopaths' annual meeting in 1997, and, following that, other homeopaths expressed their interest and support. *Homeopathic Color Remedies* was then published by the Crossing Press in 1998, and a worldwide response put these remedies out into the realm of healing. Practitioners from many different modalities in many countries have used the color remedies successfully and encouraged me to move forward with proving the sound remedies.

My thanks go to the homeopaths who did the original provings in their clinical practice: Cheryl Conran-Brown, RS Hom, and Maxine Fawcett, RS Hom, both reliable and grounded in their approach to homeopathy. The provers came from friends, patients, and interested people, to whom I am deeply grateful.

My gratitude extends to all those willing people who took the initial batch of color remedies and helped me understand that these were indeed powerful healing tools. Thanks to Dave Evans and Greg Conforth, Lakeland homeopaths in the UK, and Melissa Assilem, RS Hom, who invited a clairvoyant friend to read the energy of the remedies many years ago; we were all amazed that her awareness of the energy was completely consistent with the findings of old, established color healers.

Thanks to the following students from the School of Spiritual Homeopathy and the Institute of Life Energy Medicine, who made and participated in the homeopathic sound provings: Bill Torretti (Dip Hom Med, SSH), Mary Kehoe, Brenda Clarkson, Grace Chapman, Dr. Charlene Warner, Lynda Lee Bell (Dip Hom Med, SSH), Sarah N. Rietemeyer (Dip Hom Med, SSH), Teresa Rafael (Dip Hom Med, SSH), Hannah Walsh (Dip Hom Med, SSH), and Proving Mistress Sandra Applequist. These remedies continue to be used by students of the school and are now available from the author.

May healing be gentle, effective, and consistent with the physical laws of nature and the spiritual laws of creation. We all want medicine that is consistent with our spiritual belief. When we seek a deep, gentle, and efficient way to restore balance, we will be set right through those very things with which we are resonant.

Introduction

We experience life through color and sound. These two qualities have the ability to trigger our senses and to bring either dissonance or healing. What we see and hear reflects the world around us, and forms our ideas and clarifies our intentions. To a great degree, our perception forms the colors and tonality of the events and experiences we live with, whether depressing or uplifting. Color and sound have the potential to bring healing and balance or dissonance and chaos. Choosing what is appropriate for our well-being requires awareness and being focused on the fact that we want light, peace, and balance.

Believe it or not, color and sound also influence how we relate to others and engage with a situation. When we perceive warmth around us, we expand our sense of self and join in; if we perceive coldness, we contract to protect and isolate ourselves. Color and sound influence us greatly, and if they were taken away we would be truly lacking in opportunities to define our selves.

Throughout our lives we embrace sounds and colors without knowing how powerfully they affect us. They shape the way we think, feel, and move in the world. If you have ever made the shift from a bustling, noisy city to a quiet place in nature, you know how different you feel in these contexts. Your senses become heightened in a peaceful place, while they become dulled with too much stimulation.

Homeopathic color and sound remedies reveal the profound influence color and sound have on our being and how, when used as medicine, they can open, balance, and redress our energy at deep levels of resonance. There is a wealth of healing power in color and sound. They can stimulate, tonify, and soothe our nervous system, as well as purify and tonify our blood and endocrine system. Their vibrations, especially when assimilated into a homeopathic dilution, which we call a remedy, are extremely subtle, opening our energy field to healing and tone. They have the potential to clarify our thinking, energize our bodies, and soothe our emotions. They are the true healing tools of the future.

Enjoying color and sound is far more than an appreciation of music and beauty. We live in a sea of sound and color, and we are affected at every level. No matter how dulled our senses become from frequent overstimulation, we still define our energy fields through these arenas. And we can use their energy as medicine to heal ourselves.

When we are deprived of sound or light, as an organism, we contract and shrivel, both physically and emotionally. In parts of the planet where people are deprived of light for long periods of time, their bodily functions are actually transformed, and their habits and behavior are distinctly different. Eskimos do not become pregnant during the long, harsh winters, as their bodies are incapable of sustaining new life at the freezing temperatures and in the near darkness that they endure through the long winters. When the light returns to the Arctic tundra, along with greater warmth, life reemerges. Cycles are reestablished and pro-creation happens.

When city dwellers are bombarded by the daily din of traffic, the roar of sirens, and the clamor of people on the move, their ability to differentiate and distinguish themselves as individuals is dulled. Their sensorium becomes externally focused, and they lose their internal connection with themselves. They literally cannot hear themselves think, and, more important, cannot reflect on life. They become automatons in perpetual response mode rather than thinkers capable of unique responses to life.

We are made from the vibrations of sound and color, and every part of our being resonates with them. When our internal energy systems are out of balance, color and sound have the ability to reestablish balance and health. Light and sounds form our being, and when we die we return to that primal experience of sound and color once again.

Sound and color transform every cell in our body. They resonate with us at spiritual levels as well. When we open our higher consciousness to the heavenly spheres, we hear angels singing their praise and glory to the Creator. Many people have lost their capacity to hear these spiritual vibrations with the advent of modern machines, telephones, airplanes, and traffic, which dampen our senses and prevent us from hearing the whisper of angels in our ears. When we lose our awareness of spiritual resonance, we lose our connection to our own wise guidance.

The world of color has also become polluted with synthetic dyes, which are harsh, vibrant, and not natural. They pervert our eye's ability to see what is true. This affects how we see the natural world. If we are desensitized by what is bright and bold, then what is natural will appear washed out, dull, and faded. Natural colors will fail to appeal to our senses. We lose our grasp on reality when we are separated from what is natural, and we eventually cut ourselves off from what is ultimately sustainable and true in life.

When we can't hear birdsong or animal noises, the wind in the trees, or the roar of the ocean, our senses become deadened. This affects us physically through a weakened immune system. Surrounded by a cacophony of electronic sounds from dissonant music, cellular phones, and city traffic, our ability to fight infection, and remain resilient through challenging times is diminished. All of this threatens our ability to hear our inner voice and trust our internal perceptions. Chaos works internally to separate us from our Creator.

Today people are trying to reconnect with Self. They have rediscovered meditation and inner reflection as ways of reestablishing their internal connection to the sounds and colors that bring peace, tranquility, and inner knowing. Our sensory receptors need to reconnect with colors and sounds so we become adept at healing shattered energy systems. When we pick up emotional nuances from words that speak either lies or love, wholeness or perversity, evil or goodness, we become stronger internally and make better choices for ourselves.

As we become attuned to negativity and dissonance through inner work and healing, we find our way back to what is real and true. Healing takes time and spiritual development becomes a priority on the path to wholeness. This journey requires strength and the willingness to make our inner connections flourish so we can withstand these challenging times. Using gentle, vibrational color and sound medicine helps us find balance and reestablish inner connections.

We know innately what warms us, what attracts and what holds us; we hear it, we feel it, and we see it. Our spirits long to be attuned to real colors and true sounds that can nourish and heal us. In the discussion about the healing properties of potentized homeopathic color and sound in this book, you will undoubtedly resonate with the concepts, which your spiritual forces know to be true. Homeopathic color and sound remedies may never have been potentized into a medicine before, but the healing properties of color and sound have been with mankind from his seminal beginnings. The Bible says, "In the beginning was the Word . . . ," and if we are to accept that metaphor of Creation, we must understand that what resonates in us as goodness, beauty, and truth has been there from the beginning of time, and we are, and always have been, one with it.

Some of what is written in this book was in the first edition of *Homeopathic Color Remedies*. Since that book was written ten years ago, the remedies have been proven many times over. Since then it has been discovered that not only are the chakras involved in these remedies, but the etheric, astral, and egoic bodies also resonate with these healing forces. Color works on the etheric body, which is the energy force; sound is specific to the astral body, which is our mentality and our longings and desires; and the egoic body is the realm of pure consciousness. This information will be covered in the following chapter.

There are many new cases to share in this book, along with some innovative ways of using the remedies. In addition to new material, this book includes an Energy Assessment for the

Chakras that you can use. We still have much more to learn about both color and sound, and information comes in daily from practitioners who work with these remedies. Homeopaths and healers from around the world send their experiences with how these remedies work. You are encouraged to share your experiences as well by contacting me through www.lifeenergymedicine.com. We need to understand more about how color and sound work; as we develop, our medicine develops.

After spending fifteen years researching color remedies, I now also research sound remedies; this provides a new way of understanding vibrational healing and homeopathic principles. It's become apparent that by refining our energy fields we become more attuned to what is required for our healing. We refine our field when we use energy medicine, such as homeopathy, acupuncture, Reiki, or hands-on healing.

Do we need color to aid our energy? Do we need sound to refine our thinking capacity? What will reestablish harmony and balance in our auric field? By using these remedies temperately, we come to understand how they work. They express our innate sensitivity to energy.

The material in this book is designed to take the inquisitive and higher mind further in its exploration of how sound and color work. Here, the dynamic effects of potentized energy, in the form of homeopathic remedies, teach us about the quintessential energetic patterns of imponderable substances that have a profound effect on how we think, feel, and function.

This book presents evidence that sound and color in homeopathic potency can transform our behavior, play havoc with our dreams, and encourage our bodies and our spirits to function better; they also help us seek out our destiny. What has become evident in working with these remedies is that we are not the mechanical creatures science wants us to believe we are; rather we are spiritual beings who resonate with the joy of sound and light, responsive to vibrational healing and open to transformation at the deepest levels. Please join me on this guided tour through the land of energy, into the realm of healing and beyond to creative expression, love, and peace, where, I believe, these remedies can take us.

Thank you.

Sincerely,

Ambika Wauters
Principal of the School of Spiritual Homeopathy
Director of the Institute of Life Energy Medicine

CHAPTER ONE

What Is Homeopathy?

For those who are unfamiliar with homeopathy, it works in the realm of pure energy. It is a complete medicine that treats symptoms based on the underlying principle that "like cures like." This means that if you have a symptom—physical, mental, or emotional—you can treat it with a remedy that actually creates symptoms similar to your own. This remedy can be made from a plant, mineral, or animal substance. Such a treatment is done with miniscule amounts of the substance that created these symptoms. The substances are diluted to various degrees, according to the strength of the remedy needed. Such pure energy can penetrate our physical, emotional, and mental barriers, providing profound and often permanent healing.

All substances impact us. In proving these substances over the past 250 years, homeopaths worldwide have discovered how plant, animal, and mineral substances and imponderables affect our physical, emotional, and mental life. We know that some remedies, for instance, go straight into the emotional realm and, when they are potentized to a certain level, they can relieve grief, despondence, and fear. Other remedies go into the mental sphere, and can dispel confusion and tonify memory (which is one of the first things to go in illness). This medicine goes much deeper than any conventional medicine, which is known to only address physical symptoms.

Homeopathy treats all symptoms that reflect a derangement in our natural health, vitality, and resiliency. It can be used from childbirth through to death. It works on the physical body, as well as the mind and spirit, from the most mundane to the deepest levels of expression. Homeopathy does not mask symptoms or push them back into the organism. It stimulates the system to throw the symptoms out, and redress what is out of balance. The stronger the potency, the more the homeopathic remedy goes into the emotional and mental sphere. The lower the potency, the more likely it will affect the physical body.

Coffee provides an example of how "like cures like" works according to the basic principles of homeopathy. If you drank a strong cup of black coffee, you might develop an upset stomach, begin to sweat, have loose bowels, find yourself unable to sleep, or become irritable and aggressive. If you visited a homeopath with these coffee-induced symptoms, you might be given homeopathic coffee, in highly diluted potency, as treatment.

This remedy is made by taking one drop of strong black coffee and adding it to ten drops of alcohol and water. It is then shaken vigorously, and a drop of this dilution is taken and added to another container of ten drops of alcohol and water. A 6X remedy, for instance, describes six dilutions in ten (X stands for the Roman numeral ten) drops of solution. The higher potencies of

2ooC describe 200 dilutions in one hundred drops of solution (C stands for centesimal or 100). We have found that these remedies, known as imponderables because they cannot be seen or sensed, work best in the lower potencies. In lower potency they have fewer reactive properties and are safe to use.

THE HISTORY OF HOMEOPATHY

Homeopathy is an ancient and well-recognized form of treating illness, which Galen, a Greek physician, first discussed in the first century after Christ. Early physicians and alchemists understood homeopathy, and Samuel Hahnemann, a German physician, formally established homeopathy as a medicine at the end of the eighteenth century. Hahnemann was an inquiring genius who realized the ancient dictum of "like cures like" held up in practice. He was a great advocate of this medicine, and taught many doctors and fought pharmaceutical companies throughout his life.

Homeopathic medicine took hold in Europe, Asia, and South America and has been used as a valid form of healing in those areas for over 250 years. The royal houses of Europe have employed it for over five generations. Homeopathy has also found its way into America and has been used successfully here for many years. There is currently a resurgence of interest in homeopathy in an attempt to deal with the overwhelming cost and insidious side effects of modern medicine.

HOW HOMEOPATHY WORKS

The power of homeopathic remedies can reach through layers of suppression, be it from drugs, emotional abuse, or mental conformity, and help a person's true nature flourish. This healing brings freedom, love, and hope. It helps people move forward in their lives, and supports them in fulfilling their higher purpose in life. Homeopathic treatment does more than rid the body of physical limitations that constrict its function. It transforms the way people think about themselves by allowing more light and truth to penetrate their being.

By using imponderables, such as color and sound, which affect the core of our being, we touch soul forces. People have responded to these remedies with improved levels of health and well-being, greater happiness and joy, and more resolve to deal with the underlying problems they face. Such remedies open channels for our own sweet natures to reveal themselves.

Hahnemann's principles for prescribing and treating chronic and acute illness have not changed in over 250 years and are effective in treating all diseases, conditions, and states of emotional and mental distress. There are no harmful side effects to homeopathy, as no toxic substance is left after a series of dilutions have eliminated them from the remedy. There are, however, periods of adjustment, which homeopaths refer to as aggravation, as the person's system readapts itself to freedom, truth, and right expression. In classical homeopathy, which is my basic training as a homeopath, we use all forms of plants, animal matter, and toxic minerals to alleviate suffering. Poisons, released of their alkaline toxicity and taken up into dilution, are the mainstay of our medicine.

Light and sound are aspects of our Materia Medica; they can be used in conjunction with other homeopathic remedies without spoiling a case. They work well with acupuncture, Reiki (which addresses these energy fields), and all forms of hands-on healing.

INDIVIDUALIZED TREATMENT

People and animals respond well to homeopathic treatment because it is safe, gentle, and effective. One reason for homeopathy's success is its individualization. This means that two people who suffer from the same condition could receive different remedies based on their own unique signature of symptoms and their own way of being out of balance, even if the two people's conditions carry the same allopathic medical label.

For instance, we have 150 different headache remedies in homeopathy. One person may experience their pain on the sides of their head, another on the top, another at the back of their head—each of these patients would receive a different homeopathic remedy. Homeopathy is a very refined and highly differentiated medicine. If you took an over-the-counter remedy that addresses all headaches in general, you would get palliation (relief). Such general remedies seldom deal with the underlying cause of a headache. A homeopath will work to differentiate your symptoms in order to find the best remedy that suits your conditions, and try to alleviate the causative factors.

Another principle of homeopathy is that it does not treat labels. It treats the individual, and his or her unique symptoms are taken into consideration when prescribing a remedy. This may depend on a person's genetic predisposition, environmental factors, and often their emotional responses to events and situations. There are over thirty-five hundred homeopathic remedies to choose from in addressing a particular case, and homeopaths assess the totality of symptoms before prescribing a remedy. Homeopathy is seldom prescriptive, meaning we ask questions and find out the root cause of a problem rather than giving it a therapeutic prescription. It does require a level of self-awareness to be used efficiently.

A medicine with this level of refinement requires a person to cultivate a level of growth and self-awareness during the treatment process. Working with a homeopath allows individuals to express themselves and discuss what is and what is not working in their lives.

WHAT ARE HOMEOPATHIC COLOR AND SOUND REMEDIES?

Color and sound affect the core of our being, and we touch soul forces with these remedies. People have responded to them with improved levels of health and well-being, greater happiness and joy, and more resolve to deal with their underlying problems. Such remedies open channels for our own sweet natures to reveal themselves to us.

There are ten homeopathic color remedies, which are made by exposing colored theatrical gels and Indian silks to sunlight and water. The colors are red, orange, yellow, green, turquoise, indigo, violet, magenta, pink, and spectrum, which is made from all the colors.

Homeopathic sound remedies are made by placing tuning forks of specific musical notes over pure water in a crystal bowl and then potentizing the water. This potentization process is the same as the process described above for using coffee as a remedy. The dilutions for color remedies are 6X (six dilutions in ten drops of alcohol and water), 12C (twelve dilutions in one hundred drops of alcohol and water), and 30C (thirty dilutions in one hundred drops of alcohol and water). The sounds remedies are potentized to 6X.

Color remedies have been available to the general public since 1998, when the book *Homeopathic Color Remedies* was published. Responses from all over the world brought unusual demands for these remedies to be used in different environments and conditions. They have been used in substance abuse treatment, in veterinary practices, with austistic children, and for relief from many physical and emotional problems never foreseen when they were originally made.

Sound remedies were first created in 2004 at the School of Spiritual Homeopathy in Chicago. The students and teacher proved their effectiveness over a period of several months. They are now in clinical use.

The History and Early Provings of Color and Sound Remedies

I made the original color remedies during the winter solstice of 1989 in the Lake District of northern England. They were the result of an offhand inquiry made during a tutorial with homeopath Ian Watson. I asked how homeopathic remedies were made, and he replied that remedies could be made out of any substance on our planet. When asked if they could be made out of color, he said theoretically that was possible. Then he suggested that I try making some and see if they worked.

After Ian Watson provided the original impetus to make the first batch of color remedies, I was left wondering how to do so. Shortly after this tutorial, I had a dream in which I was shown how to make the remedies. So I gathered all the equipment I needed: distilled water, theatrical lighting gels in full spectrum colors, beakers, and small cosmetic mirrors that could be tied around the containers. Since I couldn't find any pink filters, I used a pair of pink silk tights to wrap around the containers as a source of that color.

So it was that I made the first batch of color remedies on the winter solstice—the day with the least amount of light in the northern hemisphere—December 21, 1989. Where I lived, in the north of England, there are only five hours of available light at that time of year. That day, the sky was overcast and the weather so dreary that I had no idea whether the color would be absorbed into the water, nor did I know whether the remedies would have any healing effect. I preserved the first remedies in vodka, which was the most appropriate fixative, as pure alcohol was impossible to obtain.

As I wondered how I was going to find anyone to "prove" them (validate their effectiveness), two friends from homeopathic college, Dave Evans and Greg Conforth, came to visit and asked if they could have a drop of color to test. I gave them each a drop of pink and sent them home after tea and a chat. The next day, Dave called to tell me he thought I should continue to look into these remedies. He reported that two patches of eczema in the creases of his elbows, which had persisted for a long time, suddenly disappeared overnight and, coincidentally, he had a fight with his partner, which was unusual as they shared a normally tranquil relationship.

Hahnemann said, in his treatise on homeopathic provings, that the best people for proving a remedy were those who lived together and shared the same conditions, having followed the same daily routines, eaten the same food, and drunk the same water for long periods of time. I was fortunate to have two communities near me that were willing to support the proving process. They were full of self-aware, open people who helped me discover how homeopathic color remedies worked. One was a large Buddhist community in Ulverston, in the Lake District, and the other was an Alexander Technique school in Kendall, also in the Lake District. Both produced ample volunteers for my project.

The original provings were amazing but confusing. All provers were given a single dose of a color remedy using a 30C potency. They were not told either the substance or the color. A volunteer from the Buddhist center, who had suffered from rheumatoid arthritis for forty years, was relieved from pain as a result of taking one dose of Indigo 30C. However, she immediately developed boils along the liver meridian of both legs. I realize now this resulted from detoxification of her liver, but at the time was mystified by what happened. Her detoxification followed the homeopathic rule of "healing from the top down and the inside out."

When I asked another prover, who took a dose of the same color, if anything unusual had happened to him, he told me that six women had fallen in love with him that week. I asked him whether this was part of his normal experience, and to what he attributed this experience—both good homeopathic questions. He said that he felt his confidence was extremely high while on the remedy. This same prover also dared to dive off nearby cliffs into the sea, which was something he had feared more than anything. He felt, while on the remedy, that he could do anything he wanted.

This original proving of indigo 30C led me to conclude that this remedy affected the pituitary gland. It gave people some control over their minds that could affect healing. One prover, who was a sedentary, cold woman in her fifties, suffered great emotional distress while on the remedy. She felt acutely detached and disconnected before taking the remedy, and the remedy exacerbated her symptoms. She went to her general practitioner and asked to be given drugs to alleviate her misery after taking the homeopathic remedy. These did not work because her suffering was psychological, not physical. What finally gave her relief was being massaged and touched by other people. So the solution to her suffering came from the proving.

After this I began a period of differentiating the remedies, determining how they worked and what their symptom pictures were. I investigated which colors helped certain symptoms and exacerbated others. My colleagues and I were looking to establish perceivable pictures of each remedy and each level of potency. It became clear that the 6X (six dilutions in ten drops of water) potency worked well on physical levels, 12C (twelve dilutions in one hundred drops of water) was a portal into the emotional sphere, and 30C (thirty dilutions in 100 drops of water) was a one-time remedy for many physical conditions as well as for the higher mental and emotional symptom pictures.

The provings revealed that indigo (blue) increased suffering for depressive people. The expression to "have the blues" seems to come from a deep unconscious knowledge about this color. Indigo leads to clarity of mind and detachment, improving thinking, but it also cools passions and provides mental focus. It proved to be healing for the unhappy woman mentioned earlier because it forced her to ground her energies and listen to her needs for personal contact, leading her to start having regular massages. It forced her to reach out and ask for help, something she had never done before.

After this experience, however, it was decided that the best way to test these imponderable remedies was in clinical provings. This testing period lasted for nearly eight years and helped us more fully understand color remedies. The sound remedies, which were made in 2004, were eventually proved in clinical situations also.

Students at the School of Spiritual Homeopathy initially proved the sound remedies. A group of twelve people participated in making these remedies. Sandra Applequist, a sound and vibrational healer and a student at the school, shared her tuning forks of the entire musical scale and acted as proving mistress. She muscle tested each fork to determine how many times it should be placed over the pure water when a remedy was being made.

After taking a sound remedy, each prover shared his or her experience. We were able to collate the information quickly to find each note's theme and to understand the healing nature it provided.

The provers shared many collective experiences as a group. The first sound remedy proved was the note D, which is affiliated with the sacral chakra. After everyone in the group took the remedy, which was administered in drop form, they all began to giggle, then laugh with more and more gusto; we all sat at our desks, laughing for a long while. The note D remedy had triggered the sense of joy and happiness associated with this energy center that is resonant with joy. The group bonded with one another during this first shared experience, and from that point they continued to enjoy doing the provings.

The sound remedies are distinct from the color remedies, which work on the etheric, or energy, field; rather, their affinity is to the astral body. (See chapter 3 for more information on the etheric and astral bodies.) They focus their action on longings and desires, mentality, and focus. The color remedies are more about our energy itself, whether there is enough, how it is balanced, and how to soothe, tonify, and stimulate it.

There were instant and immediate reactions to the sound remedies. They did not need time to be absorbed or to work their way into the system. As a consequence, they have never been potentized past their original potencies of 5–7X. Anyone who takes them has an immediate response, even though it may be subtle. Sound remedies do not last for very long, but they work deeply and turn around our thinking and perception quickly. We have found them to be far more potent than the color remedies and their use is distinct as well.

Differences between Color and Sound Remedy Provings

After taking the color remedies, the provers experienced a variety of symptoms. With the sound remedies, nearly everyone had the same response. They worked more collectively and less individually than the people taking color remedies. Some of the color remedies produced very clear physical characteristics, while others seemed to work more subtly on emotional and mental levels.

For instance, a very interesting thing happened to all the provers who took homeopathic color remedy pink. They all dreamed of being with their mothers, or of motherhood. These dreams were always soothing and comforting. One woman, who was pregnant and contemplating a termination, decided to go ahead with the pregnancy after taking the color. Pink was obviously about mother love, and it triggered this response in her.

The group taking sound remedies experienced collective laughter and hunger, and felt unified throughout the proving. They would stay together as a group, unable to leave one another, even if they had to go to the toilet or wanted to eat. They would walk like ducks in a row down the street, happy to be together. They were inseparable. When difficult experiences emerged in the provings, it happened to the whole group, not just to one person. It was as though the color individualized people and the sound communalized people.

The homeopathic color remedies differ from conventional color healing, which uses light and pigment applied to the skin or through the eyes, because they go deeper into a patient's energetic economy (mind, body, and spirit) and have a specific affinity with the etheric field of energy. The most obvious information learned about the colors was that they work in relation to the chakras, or energy centers of the body. These are nonanatomical energy points located in the subtle energy sheath we call the aura. The chakras channel vital energy into the physical body and act as conductors, or filters, from the etheric body.

The sound remedies act on the astral field, which lies next to the etheric field. It is the interface between the energy body and the higher mind of the Ego, or "I am" principle, that defines our individuality. The astral body is the repository of our longings, desires, thoughts, and attitudes. If these are positive, more energy flows into the etheric field and our energy is vibrant. The more negative or fear-based these are, less energy filters through into the etheric, creating depletion and lack and often leading to illness and weakness. This will be discussed more thoroughly in the following chapter.

Clinical Provings

After the initial efforts, all the color and sound remedy provings were done in clinical situations where the remedy was indicated for the patient and used to treat their symptoms. A classical homeopathic case was addressed, and the patient's physical, emotional, and mental symptoms indicated which color and/or sound remedy to chose.

Using the Energy Assessment guidelines in the back of this book can help you determine which remedy is best suited for a person. You can ask your client specific questions that indicate what chakra needs immediate healing. Then you can choose an appropriate theme for their life and choose a color or sound remedy to support their healing process.

Other ways to diagnose which sound or color remedy is required is to look at what organs are affected and the area of the body where the symptoms are located. This, along with the emotional issues a person is currently addressing in their life, can lead to discovering the blocked chakra and an appropriate remedy. We know that chakras impact the ductless glands of the body, and they, in turn, affect the system located in their area. By deciding what organs or systems are in need of healing, you also will come to the color or sound that can best treat the symptoms.

For instance, if a person is experiencing pain in their lungs or chest, green or pink would be an appropriate color remedy. The appropriate sound remedy would be F. If a person was experiencing lack of confidence, the appropriate remedy would be yellow or E, which relate to the solar plexus chakra. If a person had a headache, either indigo blue or the note A would be appropriate. Both are resonant with the brow chakra.

In every case, the color or sound remedy helped the prover in some significant way. The results indicated that the ongoing process of psychological and spiritual development can be enhanced by the use of colors and sound remedies to stimulate weakened or overactive subtle bodies and corresponding chakras. (See chapter 3 for a discussion of subtle bodies.)

It was more useful to give a color or sound remedy that was indicated by clinical diagnosis for specific symptoms than to randomly prove a sound or color in an experiential sense. For example, one redheaded prover, in the early days of provings, took red and then tried to kill her husband with a dinner fork by stabbing him in the chest. Red was not the color this already-inflamed woman needed. She would have experienced healing with the cooler colors, although we would never have known how powerful red could be on the emotions had she not taken it.

Another highly volatile prover threw all his wife's best china against a wall in a rage. He did not need the hot color of orange but rather something more soothing to sedate his fiery temperament.

It became apparent that these hot people needed cooling down, not fueling up. This was a very pragmatic way to begin, but we no longer prove remedies in this fashion. We assess what needs healing (see the Energy Assessment in the back of the book) and prescribe from that.

An example of clinical provings is as follows: A patient who experienced chronic pain from several back surgeries did well on the sound remedy of the note D. It alleviated her discomfort and gave her the energy she needed to pursue her career and live a good life.

Those who have become stuck in their lives have a strong affinity with sound remedies. Sound shifts their energy and allows them to think about their lives in a clear and focused fashion. Sound remedies work on a higher mental plane than the color remedies and seem to be directly connected to our astral forces, which control our mental processes and the way in which we think about our lives. From direct clinical experience, it has been observed that these homeopathic sound remedies bring the gift of healing.

WHAT ARE CHAKRAS?

This is an appropriate juncture to introduce the chakras. The chakras are nonanatomical energy centers that channel energy into and out of the physical body. They are the template for our health and vitality and the repository of our experiences. They are affected by the degree to which we are positive and respond well to color and sound. The amount of energy circulating in each chakra determines our level of vitality and well-being and how our physical organs and systems are functioning.

The chakras correspond to colors, sounds, emotional issues, and archetypes, and they are present in all organic life forms. They also correspond to color and sound remedies, which are similar in nature. The principle of like cures like is applicable to chakras, color, and sound. Color and sound balance and tonify the chakras and the subtle bodies (the physical, etheric, astral, and egoic bodies, which are described in chapter 3) through their vibrational resonance. The chakras are a focal point for shifting energetic and emotional blocks, and color and sound contribute to this transformation in a major way. Homeopathic color and sound remedies act as a medicine for our energy body.

I began to explore the nature of the chakras in 1990, and by 1993 I had published the first of eight books on the chakras, their emotional components, and the life issues associated with them. These books explore the nature of these energy centers and how positive thought, energy massage, and, particularly, awareness transform our energy and strengthen our chakras. The second and third books explore the archetypes of empowerment, vitality, and responsibility as they correspond to the chakras.

OFFICIALLY POTENTIZING THE COLORS: WINTER AND SUMMER ENERGY

John Morgan and his staff at Helios Pharmacy in Tunbridge Wells, Kent, England, officially potentized homeopathic color remedies in early 1992. Potentization is the process of taking the original tincture up to six, twelve, and thirty dilutions. Another batch of color remedies was made in 2004 in California, using Indian silks as the color source. They were made in bright sunlight, and they have a much stronger vibration than the original English remedies. They are the source of all homeopathic color remedies now sold.

When the remedies were first taken to Helios in 1992, there were two batches: one made at the winter solstice and another made at the summer solstice. We dowsed to see which batch had the strongest energy field. What we found was interesting. The hot colors of red, orange, and yellow were strongest in the winter solstice batch. Green, turquoise, indigo, and violet were strongest in the summer solstice batch. Nature gave her warmth when it was coldest, and her coolness when it was hottest. Magenta and spectrum were the same in both batches. We took the strongest colors from both batches and made our remedies from them.

Catherine Bolderstone, a homeopath, was the person who potentized the remedies at Helios. Since that time, she has developed a deep interest in color. She kept an account of her personal process while potentizing the remedies, and her personal journal, written during that time, reads like a fairytale. While working on the process, she met her husband, was courted, and married. Shortly thereafter, she had her first baby. The colors impacted her life, and she felt their direct influence in the events that happened to her while she made the homeopathic color remedies. She now makes color remedies of her own, using prismatic light as the source.

ADVICE ON USING HOMEOPATHIC
COLOR AND SOUND REMEDIES

The color remedies are now seventeen years old and are ready to be used by both homeopaths and the lay public. The sound remedies are three years old and just finding their way into clinical use. They are gentle, safe, and effective in treating physical, mental, and emotional symptoms. Many of the original problems encountered at the beginning have been eased with time and experience. In the beginning, I was a student, unsure of myself and not aware what I was facing. Now, I am a fully qualified homeopath with years of clinical experience behind me. As I developed my skills, working with the sound remedies has been easier and more efficient.

In the field of vibrational medicine, homeopathic color and sound remedies fit somewhere between flower essences and homeopathic plant remedies. They are similar to the flower essences, as they work to rebalance disharmonious energy states. They work best when used in conjunction with deep-acting homeopathic mineral, plant, or hormonal remedies. Color and sound remedies support the action of constitutional treatment. These remedies also work well on their own, particularly for spiritual insight and emotional harmony. There are many practitioners around the world who have had outstanding results working with the color and sound remedies by themselves, in spite of the fact that they know very little about homeopathy.

One colleague in Ireland, Monica O'Malley, has had outstanding results working with addiction, and severely handicapped children. She is a healer who works with Syntonic light therapy in addition to using the homeopathic color remedies. There are other practitioners who use just these remedies and see results.

These remedies are not meant to replace deep-acting homeopathic care or medical treatment. Many people inquire whether these remedies can cure long-standing chronic disease. They cannot do that. Please be advised that it is best to consult a homeopath or doctor regarding deep-acting and long-standing chronic diseases. Color and sound remedies work by opening an energy field so healing can happen and, in this respect, make good support remedies for other forms of deep-acting treatment. On their own, however, they are not strong enough to treat serious conditions and should never be used in this way.

Color and sound remedies easily transform energy states, such as moodiness, fatigue, exhaustion, confusion, or anger. They can be used to increase energy and to provide tonification and soothing, but cannot reverse pathology on their own. They offer support and gentle healing, and can create a positive response. Ascribing more to these remedies than they can actually do would not serve healing. We recognize that sometimes people need stronger treatment for their conditions. These remedies also support other modalities.

HEALING FORCES

By potentizing light and sound the homeopathic way, we bring the quintessential vibration of those energies into play with our bodies and spirits so they can rebalance and recharge us. Light and sound are food for our nerves, blood, and tissue, as well as for our spirits. They also free up our emotions and mental states, as we have witnessed throughout the provings. There are cases where they have transformed physical pathology, but the response is not consistent. Rather than appear cavalier about their properties, it would be wiser to suggest caution.

One of the excellent results of using these remedies is that they provide us with a model for self-awareness, helping us to understand ourselves better. By understanding the colors and the chakra system, we can see our own psychological and developmental issues more clearly. And when we see them, we have the opportunity to transform them. This helps us take greater responsibility for who we are and how we can free up our energy when it is arrested.

For instance, if we are having problems with confidence, the indicated color is yellow, which relates to the solar plexus chakra, and has to do with personal power, confidence, and self-worth. Looking at where we are limited helps us to reprogram our minds to let in more love and light, accept ourselves with unconditional love, and build grounded and real confidence in our ability to make good choices.

If we are having problems with joy, the note D is the remedy that stimulates our second chakra, which focuses on this issue. This sound remedy creates laughter and a lightness that may heal what has been heavy and serious. We can use this remedy when we wish to cultivate more joy in our lives. It helps open us to the realm of happiness and well-being.

These remedies support balance and harmony as they open doors to awareness that help us honor our worth. They encourage the subtle flow of energy through our systems and create awareness of our soul's forces and the spiritual impulses that make up our being.

When Sir Isaac Newton said, "The universe is filled with color," he could have added that it also encompasses a remarkable harmony of the spheres, which carries an eternal vibration of love and bliss. That, too, is who we are. Using these remedies helps us connect to the inner awareness that we are made of color and sound.

CHAPTER TWO

Color and Sound in the Human Energy System

Color captured the imagination of Sir Isaac Newton, one of the greatest scientific minds in history. He explored color, endeavoring to learn what it is, and his conclusions about the nature of light and its components, which we call the visible spectrum, are still honored by the scientific community today.

We owe our understanding of the fundamental properties of light to Newton, but color was understood and used in healing for thousands of years before his discoveries. We know the early Egyptians used crystals to focus color onto parts of the body for healing purposes, balancing mind, body, and spirit. They also loved sunlight and knew of its healing properties. They worshipped the sun and created healing chambers where light was directed, like today's lasers, onto the body. They understood color's physical and emotional properties, even developing some color pigments that we can no longer replicate; they also respected its esoteric aspects. Color had symbolic meaning for them, as is seen in their ancient tomb drawings.

Many peoples have also used sound as a healing agent. Tibetans have used singing bowls to heal the chakras for unknown numbers of generations. Metal alloys were blended and forged to create singing bowls (bowls that produce a warm tone when struck or stroked with a soft mallet) with perfect pitch. They knew that the proper mixture of certain metals would directly affect the chakras and open the field for healing.

Today, we are again using color and sound to reawaken our deepest potential for healing, as well as for personal growth and self-development. Color and sound can expand our consciousness, heal our wounds, and help us develop new ways of looking for solutions. They are gentle, effective, and provide us with a wonderful tool for balancing our systems.

We now have an advanced technology that allows us to break down color into energy; lasers and crystal spectography are techniques that enable us to use color more directly. We are developing the wisdom to know how to use light and sound as medicine in both allopathic and homeopathic forms that are kind to the body and loving and supportive to our being. New advances in the use of light and sound go directly into our energetic field. This book is dedicated to explaining the power of homeopathic color and sound and how they can be used for healing the human energy system.

COLOR, LIFE, AND
THE ELECTROMAGNETIC SCALE

Color is fundamental to life. Its vibrations are necessary for physical growth and healthy development. When people are deprived of light and color, they do not grow, either mentally or physically.

Color exists in the form of oscillating light waves, which, when viewed through the light spectrum, are broken down into components of white light. When we look at the energy emanations that come from cosmic rays as they enter the earth's atmosphere, we see that white light is only a small portion of a greater energy.

Modern scientists use the electromagnetic scale to measure the cosmic forces as they penetrate our earth's atmosphere. At one end of the electromagnetic scale, there are gamma rays, which may be found in the nether regions of the cosmos. These rays oscillate at a particular speed and vibrate at a fixed rate. The vibrations slow down as the rays enter the earth's atmosphere, and the gamma rays are transformed into X-rays, with their own fixed patterns of movement and vibration. As this energy slows down even more, it is transformed into ultraviolet light. In the next step of deceleration, the energy becomes white light, which further breaks down into the colors of the spectrum. As these waves of energy slow down even more, they turn into infrared waves, then microwave, radar, FM radio, television, short wave, and finally AM radio waves. The electromagnetic spectrum consists of wavelengths ranging from light to radio (sound) waves.

Sound also exists in waves and is measured by its rate of frequency and its level of vibration. We know there are sounds so low- or high-pitched that the human ear cannot register them. However, animals can register many of these sounds. When people are exposed to these extreme sounds, they can suffer from serious conditions. We want to eliminate overstimulation from both high or low sound and light frequencies.

MEASURING ENERGY WAVES WITH THE ELECTROMAGNETIC SCALE

The electromagnetic scale is measured in meters. Some electromagnetic waves, such as radio waves, are hundreds of meters long. Others, such as visible light rays, are much shorter, about 0.0000005 meter in length. An energy wave is like a rope that is continually oscillating up and down, creating peaks and troughs, and the energy vibrations are perpendicular to the direction of their propagation. Energy wavelengths reflect the distance a wave travels in one cycle of vibration, between two crests of a trough. A vibration's frequency is the number of waves that pass a point in one second. The energy, or brightness, of a wave of light is proportional to the amplitude from the crest of one trough to a zero, or center, line. White light is a mixture of many wavelengths.

As we work with the vibratory frequency and oscillation of energy waves, it is apparent that various remedial substances fall within the same vibrations as specific colors and sounds. For instance, antimonium crude and *Berberis* vulgaris are a mineral and a plant remedy, but both substances fall into the field of yellow vibrations and both resonate with the musical note E. The symptoms these plant and mineral remedies address share a psychological and physiological pattern, both with the color remedy of yellow and the musical note E. Every substance we have on earth falls into a ray of the spectrum. We can identify its ray by seeing what color the plant or mineral is, but also by what symptoms the substance addresses. For example, a remedy that works on the adrenal cortex of the kidneys will be in the orange or orange-yellow ray of light.

A mineral remedy will have a deeper and longer-lasting effect than a plant remedy, which will, in turn, last longer than a color or musical sound remedy. However, color and sound remedies help bring harmony to the mind, body, and spirit—a person's energetic economy—by virtue of their similar vibratory frequencies. How colors and sounds resonate in our body at specific frequencies is discussed in the section on chakras in chapter 3.

All medicines fit into the light-emitting energy range of the electromagnetic scale. Homeopathic color remedies, which are made from natural substances, reflect one or another color of the visible light spectrum. They also resonate with the sound remedies. All substances, or remedies, are part of the continuum of light, sound, energy, and vibration. Knowledge about this scale helps us understand the healing properties of our medicines.

CASES OF USING COLOR AND SOUND TO HEAL ENERGY

As you study the qualities that relate to each color and sound, you will begin to understand which remedies each patient needs for their healing. For example, you may see a person who appears "out of it." They hover in the realms of the cosmic forces and are not fully incarnate. This person lives in the color violet and the note of high C. They lack the red of life energy and the vibration of middle C, which is grounded. They can show pale shades of blue or violet when you look into their energy fields. There is not enough physical energy in their field. Their lower chakras are weak because they live in another realm of existence. They would do well to have the lower sound remedies and the hotter colors, which would ground their spirit and help them connect with the world around them.

Colors and sounds can be quick and effective in treating this person's energy, bringing back their natural vitality and returning them to the flow of life. These patients do well when treated with such homeopathic remedies as camphor or coca, which fit into the violet ray or high C. Using these color and sound remedies strengthens their earth forces and brings them into a space where they can relate to life more easily, as opposed to staying separate and isolated.

Giving this person the energy of violet or high C, which will exacerbate their disconnection, follows the principle of like curing like. An alternative treatment method, the traditional color healing choice, is to give them the color red or middle C, which will bring their vibration down to earth quickly. Both sets of remedies will serve their healing process, releasing tension from their upper centers and allowing their spirit to come into their body.

At other times, we see people who are too earthbound, too fired by the passions of life. They lack refinement, and their bodies are plagued with the diseases of the lower vibrations, which fall into the red or orange part of the spectrum. Their pathologies tend toward inflammatory processes, as well as poor distribution of their vital energy. When we give them hot colors, their energy is freed, allowing their higher centers of spirituality to thrive.

Again, you can give them either red and/or middle C, following the homeopathic approach, which will inflame them and burn off some of their lower vibration energy, or you can follow traditional color healing methods and give them blue or violet and/or high C, to raise their energy to a higher chakra.

All homeopathic remedies have their place on the electromagnetic scale of color and sound. We look at energy in relation to our patients' needs, to help facilitate their healing and balance. As we explore the nature of their symptoms, we can see whether their etheric forces, or chakras, need to be addressed with color or sound remedies.

Symptoms can be addressed with constitutional homeopathic remedies, herbal tinctures, or even vitamins. Constitutional remedies are specific to a person's totality of symptoms, whereas a color or sound remedy addresses the field that is out of balance and helps to create flow and vitality again where it has been arrested. Homeopathic sound and color vibrational remedies, used with other remedies or alone, help people do more than heal a symptom; they help people move forward in their life. They open the chakras so healing can happen. They are like an energetic vitamin pill for whichever chakra or subtle body needs addressing. (See chapter 3 for a full description of the four subtle bodies.)

BALANCING ENERGY UNIVERSALLY

The electromagnetic scale contains the energy we need to balance not only ourselves, but all life forms on our planet. Where a person's energy fits on this scale can give us information about what needs healing and how we can best provide that. This is where vibrational medicine becomes part of the universal energy forces. It can also be applied to animals, plants, and the environment.

As we look at what needs healing, we determine where the source of imbalance lies. If it is in a person's etheric body, we need to examine which chakra is in need of balance. If energy needs to be rejuvenated through stimulation, either a color or sound remedy is an excellent way to begin the healing process, as it opens the space for healing to happen. These remedies are so gentle they can do the job of bringing balance to the system and can also support other forms of healing.

If a person needs more cerebral energy or more spiritual insight to think about the situations in their life, then treatment should begin with a sound remedy, which encourages healing in the mental realm. In the past few years, it has been shown that the power of the mind truly plays a considerable part in whether people will heal or not.

Sound remedies clear mental stagnation, reflected in negative thought forms, which may appear as self-hatred, self-loathing, or obsessional fears that are self-limiting beliefs. A sound remedy can shift congested thought forms, help release unhealthy desires, and eliminate phobic aversions, thus allowing energy to flow into the etheric and physical bodies with more ease and clarity. As energy moves down into the etheric and physical bodies, assist it with color remedies.

As we use these energetic forces for healing, our planet's vibrational field also will move to a higher vibration. These truly are remedies for the future. However, it takes time and understanding to accept that something as ethereal as light and as simple as a musical note can affect the human energy system and our world with such a profound impact.

It is interesting that most of the remedies we use in homeopathy fall into the color range of yellow to lime green, or the musical note E. We do not need to use the lower vibrations of red and orange as often. It is also interesting to note that in healing the chakras, the energy center that needs healing the most often is the solar plexus, which resonates with the color yellow and the note E. This means many people are working on old childhood issues of loss and abandonment, seeking their center, owning their power, and trying to move into the heart chakra, where love, peace, and joy reign. This is the transition the whole planet is undergoing at this time. It is part of our collective evolution.

The solar plexus chakra deals with issues of personal power, self-worth, and confidence. Its primary focus is on knowing our worth, finding our freedom, and the right use of power. In acupuncture the solar plexus represents the fire element and relates, at a psychological level, to healing the wounds of an unloved childhood and cultivating a strong sense of Self. When we work to strengthen this chakra, we know who we are and who and what is for our highest good. As we grow in spiritual consciousness, we lay the past to rest and move forward in life with clarity about our purpose. We come to know that we are worthy of the love we say we want. We know what our value is.

On a universal level, working with this chakra is about transforming ideas of power into the reality of love. This comes when we kindle the flame of love within ourselves through healing, reflection, and meditation. In terms of vibrational medicine, this means we are moving from the brilliance of the yellow light and the note E to the neutral and soothing color of green, a color associated with the heart chakra and the musical note G. We are all dealing with this level of inner development.

CHAPTER THREE

Using Color and Sound to Heal the Chakras

Chakra *means "wheel of light."* It is a Sanskrit word describing the vortices of energy that filter the life force through the different layers of subtle bodies. They are cone-shaped in appearance, with the apex of the cone pointing in toward the body and the funnel out toward the environment. The chakras act as conductors for the electromagnetic field. This field, when fully functioning in each chakra, gives us a sense of well-being and balance. We feel in the flow of our lives as well as open and receptive. We are mentally alert, emotionally in touch, and physically resilient, with the vitality we need to meet our challenges.

At this stage in our evolution, the human energy system possesses eight major chakras and twenty-one minor chakras. (All the acupuncture points are minor chakras.) These chakras, or energy centers, filter energy into the physical body from the etheric field surrounding the physical body. This energy stimulates the endocrine system, which, in turn, release hormones into the bloodstream. These affect our growth, development, and balance, and have a profound effect on our mental and emotional well-being.

THE SUBTLE BODIES OF THE HUMAN ENERGY SYSTEM

All living things are comprised of an energy system; in humans it is called the human energy system. It is made up of several subtle bodies, or sheaths of highly refined energy. Each surrounds the body and fits into the aura, or greater outer sheath, which protects us from environmental and psychic attack. Our aura keeps our spirit intact and helps us maintain our energy field by allowing energy to flow through our system.

The aura is divided into four subtle bodies: the physical body; the etheric, or energy, body; the astral, or mental, body; and the egoic body, which is the Higher Self, or godlike aspect of our being. The subtle bodies correspond to organs of our physical body as well as to specific emotional and spiritual aspects of our personality, and they resonate with different life challenges. We study these bodies because they help us develop a clear and conscious image of how energy works, how the body and spirit function together, and how we can fulfill our destiny through coming to know ourselves in our totality. Health is a function of balance in all the subtle bodies.

The study of sound remedies has opened up a new vista in learning how the etheric, astral, and egoic bodies influence our health. This information has come from a study of anthroposophy (the study of man) and the work of Dr. Rudolf Steiner. He was a pioneer in the field of Spiritual Science, teaching how these bodies affect our nature and how to bring healing to their imbalance.

The Physical Body

The physical body deals with a person's cellular, metabolic, and systemic activities. It is our flesh and blood, bones and ligaments; in other words, it is the mineral matter of our being. It is also the vessel that holds our spirit. It is not, however, who we are or what we think and feel, no matter how much science tries to reduce our habits and behavior to biochemical reactions.

The physical body is especially influenced by (1) genetic predisposition (what we inherit from our parents and ancestors); (2) miasms (root causes of chronic diseases); and (3) our mobility and expressive patterns, which reflect our attitudes about ourselves, others, and life. These attitudes actually reflect our soul nature and resonate through all the subtle bodies.

When we address genetic predisposition in homeopathy, we look at the chronic diseases that run through a patient's life as well as in their family history. This information suggests appropriate remedies to help cleanse cellular stagnation and chronic dysfunction in the physical body. With these remedies, we can also prevent the taint of chronic diseases from being passed down to the next generation by treating people before they have children. It is one of the most profound aspects of homeopathy.

The chakras and color remedies are associated with five specific miasms: the root chakra and color red correspond to the psoric miasm, the sacral chakra and orange are related to the sycotic miasm, the solar plexus chakra and color yellow relate to the syphilitic miasm, the heart chakra and green relate to the tubercular miasm, and the throat chakra and turquoise correspond to the cancer miasm. These taints, which affect the nature of miasmic dysfunction or genetic predisposition, are found only at a cellular level, and are entrenched in a person's physical body. They are shifted only by deep-acting homeopathic remedies called nosodes, which are able to clear the miasm from the cells. These are powerful tools for healing but should be administered only by a professional homeopath.

The emotional, mental, and spiritual components to our being are connected with color and sound through the etheric, astral, and egoic sheaths. In this regard, the body has no mind of its own, but is a reflection of the higher bodies, which act as conductors for energy. The more we come to the core of our being, where we are color and sound, the more we resonate with these remedies and the more they impact our being.

Physical health allows a person to use their body to assimilate everything that is external to it, such as their physical surroundings—geology and climate—and nutrition. The body requires self-discipline and activity. It functions well when the senses are open and there is an alertness and ability to respond, with free play of the limbs and with extensive possibility of movement. Our body is the tool we use to perceive the world around us. It is also the instrument we need to fulfill our tasks on this earth plane.

Illness, according to Dr. Rudolf Steiner, educator and philosopher, can be the consequence of disinterest in the world or an inability to assimilate experiences. Illness is a form of inner disassociation, a lack of interest or desire to learn. The lesson from illness is that it teaches us about ourselves and what we need to do. The way to health becomes a function of participating in the things that give us joy and make us happy.

The physical body corresponds to the mineral kingdom and is deeply connected to the earth. Too much earth energy in a person can lead to obsession, melancholia, delirium, and inflammatory processes. Too little can lead to anxiety or excessive head activity, which can produce exhaustion, coldness, and degeneration. Keeping the body in harmony with the elements and the world around it leads to a healthy life.

Color and sound remedies can assist the body in staying strong, resilient, and flexible by adding a vibrational dimension that nourishes the energetic field, allowing more energy to flow into the physical sheath. They can also cool and soothe the body when it is overly stimulated or when there is too much energy passing through it. Health is a function of balance, which requires tonification, stimulation, and soothing in proper proportions.

The Etheric (Energy) Body

The etheric, or energy, body corresponds to the layer of vital life force energy that surrounds the physical body. It acts as a conduit for energy to work its way into the physical body, where it can be utilized for metabolism and a well-functioning body. In homeopathy this is called the vital force. The etheric body provides the fuel that drives the physical body. This life energy is channeled through the chakras, or energy centers, of the etheric sheath, or layer. These centers affect the body's organs and glands and stimulate them to release hormones into the blood.

The chakras, which correspond to physical systems, inner emotional qualities, and life issues, exist in the etheric body. They develop and become functional in seven-year periods, starting at conception and continuing through the years until they are open and fully expansive in our late forties.

The physical and etheric bodies are strongly linked. They work as a unit, with the etheric forces moving and propelling the body toward physical growth, mental development, and spiritual realization. In the etheric realm, color remedies dominate, while the sound remedies help to filter energy from the astral body (the next layer of subtle energy) to the etheric and physical bodies. Whereas work on the astral field helps us establish positive and clear thinking, work on the etheric body gives us abundant energy for our physical needs. Just attending to the needs of the physical body does not cultivate the higher centers.

The Astral (Mental) Body

The astral body is more refined and subtle than the etheric body. It works mainly with our mental processes, corresponding with sound, music, and ideas. It is directly related to our thinking, especially to our desires and aversions. Our astral body will expand or contract depending on how we think, what we like, and what we dislike. The channel for developing our thinking, it also works on our spirit.

If our thinking is strictly material, without any spiritual affinity, then our astral forces will be coarse and underdeveloped. When we begin to consider the realm of spirit and the enormous influence the spiritual hierarchies have in our lives, we start the process of cultivating our astral body. It grows as we develop. Developing clear and focused thinking expands our capacity to connect with the spiritual forces that guide our lives as well as the energy that sustains us. When our astral body is not aligned with our etheric or physical bodies, we experience a form of anxiety separation. We feel we are not connected or centered in our own being.

Sound remedies work closely with the astral body. When it is balanced, it expands and fills the etheric and physical bodies. The power of the subtle bodies is that they work together to propel us forward in life. The strength of the astral body is that when we think positive thoughts and self-affirmations, there is an abundance of energy available to us. When we think negative thoughts and lack a sense of our worth, we have little energy to work with.

The Egoic (Higher Self) Body

The egoic body is the highest part of our consciousness and defines who we are. It forms as we mature. It is that part of us that recognizes our own uniqueness, goodness, and sense of worth. When we know who we are and that we are worthy of love, kindness, and respect, we begin to develop and cultivate our egoic body. This is known in metaphysics as the "I am that I am" principle. It takes us beyond the time-space continuum into the realm of the eternal, where every positive thought and generous act becomes etched into the cosmic forces working for the good.

When we connect with this aspect of Selfhood, we experience what the Buddhists call our own true goodness. We become intimate with ourselves and retract our projections onto the world. We become responsible and self-aware and make an effort to work for the good of the world. We are no longer victims of circumstance when we know our true selves. As this subtle body develops, we learn to accept our karma and thus become empowered. The consequence of this is that the very presence of our being helps to make the world a better place. Work on the egoic forces is facilitated through meditation, reflection, and solitude.

Color and sound remedies work quickly and efficiently on people whose egoic sheath is developed. These remedies also help those in the process of developing their egoic body.

WHAT DO CHAKRAS DO?

The chakras are nonanatomical in character and exist in the etheric body. They penetrate all the other subtle bodies but work primarily in the physical body through their corresponding hormonal gland. For instance, the brow chakra is located in the area of the pituitary gland, and the throat chakra is located near the thyroid gland.

In this book the chakras are called by their English names, which correspond to their location in the physical body. Their traditional names are in Sanskrit, which may be difficult to remember, though the translation of their meaning and purpose is beautiful. For instance, in Sanskrit the sacral chakra (located in the pelvic region) is called *Svadistana*, which means "my own sweet abode."

The chakras relate to traditional Hindi gods and goddesses of folklore. Chinese, Indian, and Tibetan medicine provide a wealth of information about the different functions ancient people ascribed to the chakras. Yoga practices also refer to the chakras, and there are now many books written about them. What makes chakras interesting to us in the West is that they are the repositories of our biography; they carry our attitudes and beliefs about ourselves that define our energy field. If we believe we are worthy, our energy field will show an expanded field that is open to receiving the goodness around us. If we do not believe we are worthy, we will struggle against all odds to prove otherwise.

The archetypal qualities of each chakra are described in an upcoming section, "The Chakras: Qualities, Colors, and Sounds" and then related to corresponding physical problems and mental and emotional issues that affect each chakra. A person's chakras can be treated with constitutional homeopathic remedies, homeopathic color remedies, and flower essences to redress imbalance.

The chakras correspond to specific colors and sounds that resonate at the same energetic frequencies as they do. The sounds and colors stimulate them, which encourages healing in the psychological archetypes, emotional issues, and life challenges that correspond to each chakra. By working to heal the physical characteristics and the emotional issues surrounding an illness, we can rebalance the chakra system, dissipate congested energy, and create vitality and resiliency. Healing our minds helps the chakras; healing the chakras helps our bodies. The action of healing is from the inside out and from the top down. This is known as the Law of Cure and is universal in all forms of traditional healing.

Color and sound healing balance whichever energetic bodies are out of synch or in distress. For example, if a person suffers from a lack of confidence, which is a solar plexus issue, we use homeopathic yellow or the note E to stimulate that chakra. In doing so we encourage the chakra to expand, and with this expansion a person's sense of worth grows. This helps people feel better about themselves and go forward in life doing positive things for themselves and others.

This is similar to acupuncture, which stimulates the points on a particular meridian in the body to increase the charge to the area deficient in energy. When the physical area is stimulated, psychological and emotional areas are also charged.

As opposed to the previous example, when people are too deeply steeped in issues of personal power, also a function of the solar plexus, they may surround themselves with too much yellow. You may notice they wear it, paint their favorite rooms that color, and even drive a car that color. Too much yellow means the egoic forces are too strong, and they need a complementary color to bring balance into their lives. The complement of yellow is violet, the color of spirituality. Giving violet to a person with an inflated ego, to wear or to take as a remedy, helps reduce their inflated ego forces and releases rigid energy, which can become fixated in the energy system. In nature, yellow blossoms are offset with violet and purple. The colors support one another, as they do in the field of the human energy system.

Blocked energy can be shifted by chakra massage (refer to my book *Healing with the Energy of the Chakras*, Crossing Press, 1993), reflective meditation, and appropriate affirmations. Cultivating a positive sense of one's worth is essential. Knowing that you are worthy of the love you seek and the things you want in life strengthens the chakras and creates a resonant field, so that what you long for materializes in your life. Chakras are attuned to positive thought forms.

It is always best to seek ways of healing that offer deep-acting transformation without being either invasive or aggressive. Homeopathic sound and color remedies provide a gentle, safe, and effective way of transforming life energy when it is stagnant or blocked. They work to address the centers and do not have either aggravation or strong detoxification effects.

The chakras are made of subtle etheric energy, and their function is to filter life energy in and out of the body, from the most substantial form of energy needed for our everyday survival to more refined levels of mental and spiritual energy.

Chakras are formed, healed, or destroyed as the life force melds itself into forms that resonate with our belief system. If we are contracted, closed, and intense, our chakras will display the same qualities and be unable to perform their function. If we are open, expansive, and loving, our chakra system will be the same and energy will be abundant and flowing.

If they are out of balance, chakras can be healed through positive thought, conscious and alert movement, and touch. However, sustaining the high vibration necessary to change old existing attitudes or patterns may require persistent efforts on our part for many years. It may require therapy, healing, and homeopathy to transform old patterns that limit our belief in ourselves. Sound and color remedies, along with flower essences, are good tools for transforming old problems that linger in our energy centers.

Color and sound remedies can increase a chakra's power and energy and help it regain cohesion and function if there is congestion or weakness. These remedies work well after trauma, injury, or separation, as they help create a unified field. When color or sound is homeopathically potentized, it acts as an energetic stimulant to the chakra and helps it regain balance and harmony to continue its job of filtering energy into the physical body.

Since a homeopathic color or sound remedy is pure energy, it is also easily assimilated into the chakra itself. When we can assimilate energy easily, we can find our balance easily. When a chakra is overcharged and drains energy from other centers, then the complementary color is best indicated. For instance, a person exhibiting symptoms of an overcharged sacral chakra—high anxiety, overeating, and frenetic activity—would need indigo to reduce this drain and stabilize the chakra. The complementary color balances the chakra and provides an energy source for the weaker chakras so harmony can be restored in the system.

Using color and sound remedies helps a person resolve physical problems and emotional and mental issues without great struggle or despair. Balance is experienced as well-being, inner harmony, and what in homeopathy is called "being well in oneself."

UNDERSTANDING HOW THE CHAKRAS WORK

Understanding how the chakras work can help us find suitable remedies to bring ease and a deeper sense of comfort to people. Since the chakras are an energetic system, homeopathic colors and sound remedies support healing at subtle levels, as well as in the more obvious physical arenas of life. When function is regained at one level, it restores balance and harmony, stopping an energetic leak at another level. Bringing healing to one chakra helps restore balance in the whole energetic system.

Time and again, both with traditional homeopathic treatment and with color and sound remedies, healing happens in both physically measurable ways and in subtle and intangible ways that cannot be measured other than through feelings of well-being and optimal function. Balance is experienced as right action and is reflected in wholesome choices for how we live and manage our energy. This allows people to move forward into a more creative and healthy way of living when their energy is whole and flowing in the proper channels. Here is a chart of the chakras and their locations, as well as a chart showing the relationships between the color and sound remedies, glands, and corresponding life issues.

THE CHAKRAS	LOCATION
Root Chakra	At the base of the spine in the perineum
Sacral Chakra	Two inches below the navel and two inches into the body
Solar Plexus Chakra	At the nerve ganglion under the sternum and over the stomach area
Heart Chakra	Over the chest, slightly to right of center, to balance the physical heart
Throat Chakra	In and over the throat area, including the mouth, jaw, and ears
Brow Chakra	Over the pituitary gland between the brows
Crown Chakra	At the crown of the skull
Alta Major Chakra	About ten inches above the crown of the head

COLOR & SOUND / GLAND	LIFE ISSUES
Red, middle C **Adrenal cortex**	Survival, grounding, organization
Orange, D **Ovaries and testes**	Pleasure, sexuality, abundance, well-being
Yellow, E **Pancreas**	Worth, esteem, confidence, personal power, freedom of choice
Green and pink, F **Thymus**	Community, nature, love, family, friendship, purity, innocence
Turquoise, G **Thyroid**	Truth, willpower, creativity, self-expression
Indigo, A **Pituitary**	Wisdom, knowledge, imagination, intuition, discernment
Violet, B **Pineal**	Beauty, harmony, spirituality, love of God
Magenta, high C **Pineal**	Preincarnation contracts, the collective unconscious, highest levels of creativity

FOLLOWING THE FLOW OF ENERGY
THROUGH THE CHAKRAS

Energy flows freely from the cosmos and enters the human energy system at the crown chakra. It also comes up from the core of the earth and enters at the root chakra. A vortex is formed where these two streams of energy meet. It acts as a funnel for energy, creating the electromagnetic field in and around the body.

This energy flows throughout our subtle bodies while we are alive. It has a dynamic movement and is constantly circulating through us. When a person dies, this energy flow ceases. The chakra itself is the conduit of the life force; it filters energy into and out of the physical body. After death it fades away until the subtle bodies have completely dissolved.

The chakras constantly filter the energy flowing through our bodies. When energy becomes stagnant, such as when a person's spiritual forces are not developed or the person has no sense of who they are or their own innate worth, then chronic illness can occur. Stagnation can trigger miasms, which is our genetic predisposition and the root of chronic disease. Homeopathy helps to clear our miasms, and it furthers our self-development and self-actualization; it helps enhance our self-love, and cultivates compassion for our suffering. It helps heal our chakras, which continue to grow and expand as we grow internally.

A block in one chakra, which may result from a limited belief or a pattern of arrested development, limits the flow of energy moving in and out of the other chakras. This will affect the entire energy body. Such limitations are experienced as weakness, malaise, low energy, self-doubt, fear, and anxiety. These limitations, along with long-term dysfunction, allow disease to take over.

If, for instance, an excessive amount of energy is flowing in and around the solar plexus, the higher and lower chakras will be weakened, which can result in massive egotism and an ungrounded sense of reality. The ego will become strong based on an inflated sense of itself. The chakra above, which is the heart chakra (or love center), will be underdeveloped because relationships would not be considered as important as self-aggrandizement. This person would place money or power before love and intimacy.

In this scenario, it is likely that the root chakra would be weak, with a limited sense of reality, and the sacral chakra would be overly expanded, with a sense of greed or gluttony.

When a relationship is based solely on a desire for self-aggrandizement rather than deep, intimate connection, the heart chakra shrinks and the solar plexus expands. This reflects a person who tries to be more than they actually are, focusing on issues of personal power and manipulation, often at the expense of others. The etiology of this in early childhood is not feeling loved and having to create a false sense of one's self to survive.

In another example, someone blocked at the throat chakra would have an overly full heart chakra and a weak brow chakra. This person would be very sensitive to emotional pain. This could manifest as having an inability to express their personal feelings, having limited ideas about themselves, and being unable to think wisely about who they are and what they are doing in life. This energetic pattern is often found in creative people and in many healers. Energy is blocked in the heart and those deep feelings cannot reach the throat to find expression. The flow of energy to the brow chakra is weak, and, as a result, clear and effective thinking and self-reflection is limited.

The flow of energy to the physical body becomes limited when either the sacral or root chakra is blocked. If issues of belonging, connection, pleasure, and well-being are not reconciled in a wholesome way, then energy becomes stagnant in these lower centers. As a result, the physical body can become weak or age prematurely.

Each chakra is supplied energy for its own particular function. The energy varies in terms of quality and quantity. However, it is the same flow of energy that comes from the heavenly and earthly forces. Each chakra needs to perform its own function, and it is dysfunctional for one energy center to do the work of another. Systemic problems arise when one center is robbed of the energy it needs in order to support an adjacent blocked chakra. It is not appropriate, for instance, for personal power to replace our need for well-being and pleasure.

Just as certain boundaries in life serve to enhance social organization and protect our individual sense of Self, so boundaries in the human energy system serve to allow each chakra to do its job in a well-defined way. Each boundary helps differentiate one energy center from another. Emergency compensation can help a center repair itself, but the long-term effects of this will weaken the totality of the system.

For example, when a person uses their sexuality (a sacral chakra function) to enhance personal power (a solar plexus function), it reflects a deep dysfunction, and eventually physical pathology of some sort will materialize in this lower center, such as in the reproductive system. Homeopathic color and sound remedies, such as orange or the note D, can strengthen the sense of ease and enjoyment and take pressure off the reproductive organs, and yellow or E can strengthen the solar plexus and develop a healthy, functioning sense of selfhood.

People who are unable to express themselves appropriately (a throat chakra issue) may have a very strong or overcharged heart chakra. They use their heart center to contain the love they find difficult to express to others. They may tire easily and suffer from weak hearts in later years. They can use turquoise or the homeopathic sound remedy G to strengthen their throat chakra and green and pink or F to strengthen their heart chakra when they feel drained. Psychologically, these people need to create relationships where they can express their love fully.

We are always working with the totality of our being, which helps us to realize we are capable of more than our limited ways of coping and managing in our daily lives. People who are confined to only one way of coping or operating in the world may need to examine what is blocked in their lives that creates an inflexible and rigid energy field. If identifying with a particular way of being, such as being a healer or homeopath, a businessperson, a teacher, or a priest, is our only way of expressing ourselves in the world, we need to see what other function is weakened and put some light (that is, color or sound) into that area of our lives.

These vibrations can help us expand our sense of life and enjoyment. Being too strongly identified with a particular way of being limits us and dampens our energy field. It creates a rigidity in our energy centers. Being more flexible in our thinking, less critical, and slower to judge others may create a more flexible and viable energy system as well.

A thought form or attitude about joy, ease, pleasure, or creative expression may need to be transformed for healing to happen in our chakras. Using color and sound remedies can open a channel for personal transformation. Color helps replenish a low energy supply so that the work of re-evaluating our lives is easier and more joyful. Sound helps us make clearer choices as we think about what and who is best for us.

As energy flows into the chakras, it stimulates the ductless glands associated with them. The stimulation of the gland releases hormones into the bloodstream and affects our health and well-being. It also opens blockages. This, in turn, feeds the body's organs and tissues, stabilizes the emotions, and helps, ultimately, to fulfill each individual's divine potential. Chakras, like homeopathic remedies, function in a broad spectrum, spanning the breadth of physical and emotional development on to the reaches of karmic destiny and spiritual growth. When we add color or sound to a chakra, we increase the intensity of vibration in that center, which stimulates the energy moving in and through the entire energy body. This has a powerful effect on a chakra's functioning. Potentized remedies have the advantage of lasting longer than direct applications, and they are easier to repeat.

For instance, when a person is in the midst of emotional separation from their partner, the heart chakra becomes weakened. We may call this grief a form of energetic starvation. The heart chakra loses its tonicity as external input of energy (from the relationship) ceases to be a sustaining element in this person's life. When this happens, the solar plexus chakra takes over temporarily to help this person rebuild their confidence and regain a stronger sense of their personal power and self-worth.

Through self-actualization, the internal mechanism of loving one's self creates energy that nourishes the heart. Eventually the heart center, which has had time to heal, becomes capable of functioning again, and love flows in and out of this chakra, becoming its sustaining force again. The locus of power here has shifted from external sustainability to internal sustainability, which not only brings healing but intensifies the quality of their energetic field.

TRADITIONAL COLOR HEALING AND HOMEOPATHIC COLOR REMEDIES

Color can be applied to the human energy system through the use of colored lights or colored clothing, eating certain foods, direct application of color to the eye, or inner visualization techniques. Homeopathic color and sound remedies are given in pill form, and are taken orally.

In addition to general color light healing, homeopathic color remedies directly influence the chakras for a substantial length of time, both stimulating and balancing the whole energetic system. Depending upon a color's potency, the length of time required for healing will vary. Low potencies will need to be repeated more often than higher ones. They can be repeated three to five times a day. Higher potencies will stay in the system longer than low ones. A 30C potency can last for weeks before needing to be repeated. It depends entirely on how depleted the chakra is of energy. If it is greatly depleted, the remedy will need to be repeated twice daily or every day. If the chakra can hold color on its own, it may not be repeated more than once. Dosages are at the discretion of the practitioner. Color remedies increase the flow of energy in a chakra, and work physically, emotionally, and mentally during the time they are active. When the old symptoms return—although to a lesser degree than their original strength—it's best to repeat the remedy.

We know from provings that color and sound remedies have a direct effect on body temperature and fluid retention; they can increase or release irritability and promote tranquility or create irritability. They assist with expressing emotions and enhancing levels of confidence and self-worth, and they influence feelings of love and hate. Depending on the potency and color, remedies can restore vitality and joy. They directly affect energy levels in people who were completely exhausted and shut down from chronic and even terminal disease. When given the color remedies, these patients made a remarkable shift on all levels of their being.

Orange 6X and Saccharine officianalis 30X have been used for deep depression in suicidal patients. These remedies revived the patients' energy and spirit almost immediately. This has become a prescriptive formula for deeply depressed patients who are unable to make healthy decisions or positive moves in their lives, and whose energetic systems are almost completely shut down.

TRADITIONAL SOUND HEALING AND HOMEOPATHIC SOUND REMEDIES

We have known from ancient times that sound—be it the use of bells, singing bowls, chanting, or toning—has a profound healing effect on our energy. Music is one of the most evocative and powerful forms of stimulation, relaxation, and rejuvenation that we have. Specific types of music, such as Indian ragas and Native American chanting, can alter our consciousness.

Homeopathic sound remedies consist of potentized notes of the musical scale that resonate with their specific chakra and directly influence the energy field related to it. The notes clarify the mind and transform our attitudes about ourselves. The sound remedies heal at a profound level by clarifying our perceptions of the world within and around us. Strengthening the astral body, which influences our emotions, and working on our aversions and desires helps clarify our sense of our right to happiness, well-being, and joy.

Sound remedies can stimulate deep levels of joy and laughter, release anxiety and a sense of separation, and help us form clear speech and profound thought. They tone the mind, helping us find ease and pleasure, and deepen our inner knowing and receptivity to spiritual guidance and protection.

Sound remedies can be used in conjunction with homeopathic color remedies or as individual remedies on their own. They are kept purposefully at a low potency because they are very strong and powerful. At this point in their evolution, they do not need further potentization.

SYMPTOMS AND THE SUBTLE ENERGY SYSTEM

It is vital for a practitioner to understand that when a patient complains about certain emotional or physical problems, the person is alluding to an imbalance in their subtle energy system. For example, we know that pain refers to an imbalance in the astral forces, and low energy or vitality refers to an imbalance in the etheric forces.

As we look for the basis of a person's health problems, it is essential to find out what they are experiencing on the emotional level. The Energy Assessment in this book reviews each chakra to help determine where a patient is functional or dysfunctional. If we look at personal problems as a causative factor in a patient's life, without recognizing that each person creates their reality by virtue of their attitudes or thoughts, we are doing our patients (and ourselves) a serious injustice. By not helping them take responsibility for their destiny, we are limiting their ability to expand their inner development and spiritual growth. Encouraging a person to come out of the victim archetype and learn to unconditionally love themselves, for example, is what homeopathic healing can offer.

When we address a person's problems and overcompensatory tendencies, we help them value their own truth in honesty and integrity. This can assist them in making healthy decisions for themselves, such as where they want to go and what they hope to do to fulfill their highest potential. We are, in effect, serving their higher consciousness (the egoic body). External circumstances can seldom be changed, but attitudes about experiences can. By changing the way we think about a situation, we release ourselves from its ties and get closer to living in freedom and love.

It lightens the burden on practitioner and client alike to come to this level of truth. This way, we literally shine light on dark areas of our unconscious and bring insight and healing into our lives. We act as facilitators when we show our patients where we see blocks and support them with the appropriate remedy to shift the balance in them from suffering to health.

Unearthing Emotional Issues Related to the Chakras

Each chakra in the etheric body focuses on a different level of emotional expression when facing different life issues and challenges at the various stages of development. This provides us with a hierarchy of awareness that helps us see individuality and personal empowerment emerge in terms of sustained physical vitality, deepening emotional truth, and the capacity to meet challenges in a mature and consistent manner.

Chakras develop throughout our lives. As we grow internally, so do they; as we become more physically present, our chakras become more resilient. The first three chakras (root, sacral, and solar plexus) are formed during the first twenty-one years of life. If they remain underdeveloped, certain healing work will need to be done to expand them to increase that person's physical vitality, enhance their personal empowerment, and strengthen their emotional well-being.

For instance, an arrested development of personal power and a failure to experience who a person truly is suggests a weakness in the solar plexus chakra. We will likely see a lack of confidence or self-esteem; ideally, this would have formed in youth, but unfortunately, the individual lacked unconditional love or a proper education to nurture a sense of well-being and self-identity. This person does not know their heart's true desire, nor do they know who they are at a core level.

Such a person often turns out to be the victim of power plays or manipulation or sometimes they may become very manipulative themselves to compensate. This may be overtly evident in a weak or impaired personality with an inability to stand up for themselves. They may look like children well into their adulthood.

From their stories, we can discern the damage to the first three chakras. They may be plagued with irrational fears, be afraid to express themselves, or have phobias or obsessions that mask their fundamental weakness and lack of strength.

People with damage to their first three chakras may also be hateful or resentful, and intense negative emotions may block their personal power. If this remains a chronic state and the person cannot break free of their limitations, they will fail to grow and thrive. We will eventually see pathology express itself in an underfunctioning digestive system, such as poor assimilation, liver problems, and gallstones. We could see diseases in the liver, the seat of anger, or in the gallbladder, where timidity about love is reflected and where frustrations can fester and solidify into stones.

If such problems are treated allopathically and steroids are administered, then a slow and steady deterioration is predicted, as a person became less and less capable of harnessing their inner resources to deal with the world, both physically and mentally. They would not find the energy to face their emotional challenges and might turn to antidepressants or recreational drugs. Allopathic drugs create so much weakness that people are left bereft, weakened, and incapable of harnessing their strength. This is a problem that healers and doctors see every day.

Instead, there are homeopathic remedies that address these problems and their pathology. There is a direct correlation between the colors and sounds and the homeopathic remedies used. These can be found at the back of the book. Reliance on allopathic medication is a diminishing return in terms of vitality, insight, and holistic treatment.

It is important to look at the energetic and emotional causative factors in any case where there is imbalance. If we treat only a patient's pathology without looking at the deeper underlying issues, we are not helping them in the long run; we are merely providing a quick fix for their problems. We may even be suppressing their physical symptoms with a treatment that does not consider the more serious underlying emotional and mental issues.

In our example of a solar plexus chakra imbalance, homeopathic healing can strengthen the patient's inner psychological state, as well as the chakra, by reinforcing egoic strength. Color or sound remedies can do this energetically, directly stimulating the solar plexus and thus increasing the flow of energy through the chakra into the ductless gland, in this case, the pancreas, which in metaphysics is known as the seat of joy.

Other homeopathic remedies address the underlying weakness as well. Sound, color, and deeper-acting homeopathic remedies stimulate digestion at both the physical and emotional levels. Homeopathy offers the choice of working at many levels to help the patient through their difficulties. However, the remedies must have a parallel resonance with the patient's body, mind, and spirit.

Following the Law of Cure, balance first reappears at the mental and emotional levels, as people gain greater self-confidence and faith in their ability to get on with their life. They begin to live the kind of life they wish for and become stronger in creating healthy boundaries, standing up for themselves, and saying no to what does not work for them.

Healing then moves into the physical arena, and the pathology begins to disappear. Physical pathology begins to clear when the egoic and astral forces are reconciled and can channel sufficient energy through the etheric body to heal the physical body.

We have seen in the provings that color and sound remedies transform the energy of underfunctioning chakras and help heal emotional as well as physical dysfunction. Throughout all the provings, patients repeatedly made statements that they were "better able to cope" and "stronger in myself." This signifies that their chakras and their subtle bodies were more functional, and the patients had more control over how they used their energy.

Emotions are not the only cause of physical distress, but they do play a very large part in the healing process. There are often hidden issues in a person's life that are deeply rooted in their energetic and subtle bodies. These become triggered by stress and then appear on the surface as symptoms.

Emotional issues come up to be healed, and it is a great sign of healing when emotions that have been deeply suppressed begin to surface. It is a sign that the vital force is reanimated. In homeopathy, our philosophy is "better out than in." We want physical and psychical toxins released from the field. That gives tranquility to the physical and subtle bodies; then healing can happen.

Healing Ungroundedness in the Root Chakra with Color and Sound

If people are ungrounded and disconnected from the realities of their physical life, this is reflected in their energy system. This ungroundedness will show up as a lack of vital heat in their metabolism, which we would see as red and orange light. They will lack strong, vital energy in their lower chakras, and their other centers will appear weak and depleted.

They may either shun the colors and sounds that are associated with these chakras or they will have a strong desire for them. Their desire for these colors is how they compensate for their energetic depletion.

Often by asking people which colors they like and dislike we can determine which chakras are in need of treatment. Asking about the emotional issues that correspond to these chakras can confirm a diagnosis; in most cases, the colors and related qualities are identical.

Healing can be administered in the form of a homeopathic color or sound remedy. The potencies range from 6X to 30C. Depending upon the patient's degree of disconnection and separation, the remedy they will need can be repeated over a period of time. As the color or sound remedy is ingested into the system, it stimulates the chakras that correspond to the color and musical note remedy, and it creates a resonant field where healing takes place.

As the person's energy becomes more balanced, they will need less stimulation and fewer doses of the color or sound remedy. This is an indication that the remedy is working and healing is under way.

The patient's emotional behavior will indicate when their chakra has been stimulated. This is true with both color and sound remedies. The patient may show signs of irritation, anger, or frustration, or may suddenly appear more relaxed, at ease, or empathic and understanding. They may develop a stronger appetite for more earthy things, such as food, exercise, sex, or material items. Irritability is a life sign and one of the signs that the system is awakening or coming out of its anesthetic state of passivity. This should not be suppressed.

If an ungrounded person, who had little interest in food, suddenly develops a strong appetite, it indicates the remedy is working. Patience, order, stability, a concern for physical security, and a desire to make their dreams come true are also signs of grounding. These are aspects of the root chakra and are associated with a strong vital force. Anger could also be a symptom that indicates they are becoming grounded.

The issues related to each chakra and the color and sound that correspond with them are given in the charts at the end of this book. Grounding and survival, as well as family or tribal issues, are related to the root chakra, whose color remedy is red and sound remedy is the note C. When a person is tired and worn out, orange or D are the remedies to consider. These work on the sacral chakra and help with rejuvenating physical energy.

These therapeutics are guided by emotional issues, and the color or sound remedy is administered accordingly. It is a simple and easy system to follow, neither complicated nor complex. It moves beyond the general physical symptoms and becomes anchored in life issues and developmental stages in an individual's life. However, it does require that the practitioner be attuned to the emotional reality of their patient.

Since we are constantly evolving and growing, we may need different sound and color remedies at different stages of our life. Classical homeopathy prescribes a constitutional remedy, which is an individual's signature remedy. With color and sound remedies, we can use the entire color spectrum or musical scale, depending on what needs to be addressed in a person's energy system. There is no one remedy as in classical homeopathy; there are many, which can be used at different times, to deal with different challenges.

We can facilitate the process of change and transformation when we acknowledge our emotional truths and take responsibility for ourselves. If we suppress and deny our issues, then we will become susceptible to physical pathology. Suppression ages us and makes our energy stagnant. When we become physically ill, it is difficult to sort out our emotions, which, by the time we are facing physical crisis, may be confused and entangled. Staying in touch with our feelings is important. This connection is a barometer for our responses to life around us.

Transforming Limited Beliefs and Attitudes

Every day in private homeopathic practices, people seek help for deteriorated health. They are often very unhappy about some aspect of their lives. And they often subscribe to the victim archetype by not doing what they want with their lives, afraid to explore the realm of possibilities that can give them happiness and satisfaction. They are stuck, fixed in a pattern of limited self-belief. They are also fixed in an archetypal response to situations they feel they cannot or will not change.

Their energy levels may be as low as their spirits. They are out of balance and out of alignment with their destiny. And their personal colors may be dark, dull, and generally unhealthy.

When you hear people say that they will wear only a certain color and would never consider another, you know they are limited in their beliefs. What is it that they get from this one color?

When they say a certain color makes them feel anxious or fearful, you know that they are unwilling to make a life change. This is an indication of blocked energy. The same is true about choices in music. What is it that we seek in sad music? In any music that we listen to repeatedly? Are we soothed or satiated by these sounds? There are so many responses to music—it is important to be aware how it affects us.

Exploring the attitudes and archetypes affiliated with the chakras helps people open up to the realm of possibilities for how they can transform their lives. Using color and sound remedies changes both a person's inner and outer vibrations, bringing healing to negative and fixed attitudes and beliefs. One of the things we witness when people begin to heal is a shift in the way they look at color and sound. Their choices for both expand and become more balanced.

SPECIFIC CASES FOR USING COLOR AND SOUND REMEDIES TO HEAL DAMAGED CHAKRAS

There are times when a chakra may be particularly damaged and need stimulation from a color or sound remedy to help establish balance. For instance, if there have been complications during a pregnancy and the baby did not receive sufficient oxygen, resultant physical symptoms may include idiocy, blindness, and impaired sensory and motor function. This means that the higher chakras, which provide intellectual and spiritual energy to that being, are impaired.

Using color and sound remedies from early in infancy can stimulate the baby's energetic centers and help repair damage, influencing the field so the energy centers become more functional. Where there is permanent physical damage, the chakras can still be stimulated to develop, and inner growth and development can proceed.

Although a child may be physically blind, it doesn't mean that he or she has to suffer emotional or spiritual blindness. Color and sound can be used to stimulate the subtle bodies of the etheric and astral forces. Building strong subtle bodies keeps a child's spirit whole and intact. This has proven to be effective in treating both physically handicapped and autistic children.

Potentized color can feed the refined energy of the higher chakras. It can nourish deprived areas of the brain and help with glandular function, motor development, and emotional and spiritual growth. Color and sound remedies have been used with many people with physical impairments, and the results over time have been beneficial, strengthening, and vitalizing.

Recently, a baby born without a thyroid gland was treated with homeopathic color remedies. She is taking allopathic thyroxin and homeopathic Thyroidinium and baryta carbonicum. She has responded well to a homeopathic color remedy of turquoise 3X (relating to the throat chakra), repeated daily over a period of months.

This infant communicates in an interesting way. She used to cry loudly and with great force when she wanted feeding or attention. After the turquoise remedy, she became less aggressive in her communication. She cried, of course, but in a different way, with less of a sense of desperation. She became confident of getting what she wanted. It no longer took all her energy to communicate her needs. After the remedy, she had extra energy for playing and was more open and direct in her communication with people around her. The color strengthened something in her life force.

Another exceptional case is of an adolescent girl with congenitally weakened kidneys. She was sexually abused as a child and was given repeated doses of antibiotics for relief of kidney infections. Her kidneys were weakened from overuse of drugs, and she continued to suffer from chronic cystitis. She responded well to staphisagria 200 and *Berberis* tincture. She also was given orange 6X to take when she felt low on energy. This gave her strength and a renewed sense of vitality. The color remedy had a direct effect on her kidneys. She has had no further infections or any reported cases of cystitis since taking the orange remedy.

The sacral chakra, whose color is orange, feeds energy into the adrenal cortex of the kidneys. This chakra governs how we respond to sexuality, finances, pleasure, and issues of well-being. As this girl improved in her physical health, she also underwent a shift in the way she responded to men. She is no longer as eager to give herself to anyone who shows an interest in her. She is more discerning and less of a pleaser. Her pathology, at an emotional and physical level, has been transformed. She is also more conscious of her self-worth.

A mentally handicapped child who suffered from seizures was given homeopathic indigo blue (related to the brow chakra). She responded well to it and deeper-acting homeopathic constitutional treatment, and her seizures diminished in regularity: she went from three to five seizures a day to five weeks without a single episode. Homeopathic indigo and the note A strengthened her ability to carry on with her tasks with more mental clarity and alacrity.

A twenty-nine-year-old man with cerebral palsy who could not speak, could not walk without crutches, and had suffered abuse in institutional care for most of his life, experienced remarkable changes while on orange, green, and pink.

The orange (sacral chakra) worked on his physical vitality, and the green and pink (heart chakra) helped his heart. He wanted to die when the case was first taken and was predicting his death. Since treatment, he no longer speaks of death, and he has straightened his spine, relaxed the tension in his feet, grown two inches, and is attempting to walk without crutches. Color had a profound effect on his gray and bleak outlook on life and gave his spirits a big lift.

A desperate woman, with neither money nor any serious prospects of earning what she needed to meet her financial obligations, was given the chord, or all musical notes. She needed to think about her challenging situation and make some healthy moves for her well-being which would support her desire to be a healer. After taking the remedy, she felt more supported in her efforts and less stressed about the challenges in her life. She was better able to think of a wholesome solution to her bind and find her way forward.

Color and sound remedies work to support people in meeting the challenges of their lives. They can provide both physical energy to go forward and mental clarity to think about situations that drain and deplete our forces, thus holding us back. These remedies have been used to bring real support through physical, emotional, and mental crises.

Two Patients with Similar Symptoms
Needing Different Color Remedies

A few years ago, two patients arrived at my clinic on the same day with exactly the same symptoms. They both were complaining of stomach cramps. One woman was a spiritual devotee of an Indian guru. This man was the master to whom she declared total surrender and obedience. She abstained from many physical and material comforts. She was also unable to look after herself properly. She lost things easily and wasn't aware of her physical surroundings. She was ungrounded and disconnected from life and required red, the color of earth and physical energy. This was also the one color to which she was completely averse.

She was given one dose of red 30, and within minutes her cramps disappeared and she appeared more connected to people and her environment. Her lack of focus and disconnection were gone. Suddenly, she was present and in her body. Within a few minutes, she became angry and wept about the lack of warmth in her life. Some time later, she became sexual again, after years of abstinence, and she continued to be more present in her experiences with those around her. Eventually, she stopped her devotion to her teacher and began doing things to support her community and her family.

The second patient was a seventeen-year-old girl who came to the clinic complaining of the same symptoms. She was in severe conflict with her mother, who was both mentally unbalanced and neglectful. This girl needed spiritual understanding in order to manage her situation. She was given Magenta 30, the opposite end of the visible spectrum from red. This is the color of the collective unconscious and spiritual acceptance.

This young girl needed a larger vision of her life in order to come to grips with her circumstances and unhappy situation. The remedy took away all her physical complaints, and she had a dream that night that helped her see her relationship with her mother more clearly. Within weeks she went to live with her father and began to study and make plans for her life, which she had been unable to do while in constant conflict with her mother. She was later given a homeopathic remedy that was deeper-acting and addressed some of her other problems, but it was the magenta that opened the door to her life as an adult.

With these two patients, colors were given according to each individual's emotional and energetic needs, not their physical symptoms. Though they were treated with different colors, their physical symptoms manifested in their solar plexus chakra. One needed insight and the other needed grounding. For deep healing to occur, we need to capture the essence of a person's inner reality.

Two Patients with Different Symptoms Needing Similar Sound Remedies

A woman who was raised in Europe came to the clinic complaining of feeling cold, disconnected, and out of touch with her family. For the last twenty-five years she had lived in the U.S. and had settled down, married, and worked for many years in social work. Her primary complaint was that she didn't feel connected. It was a cold winter that year, and her neighbors were all blockaded in their homes. She struggled with the long winter without the respite of a holiday break. She was given the musical note middle C, and within a short period of time her sense of being connected—with herself, her family, and her community—revived. This remedy helped her focus her thinking on the good things around her, and she again felt connected to her home and her neighborhood. She began visiting people and reaching out after the sound remedy.

In another case, a woman who suffered from severe lower back problems and occasional depression did well on the musical note D. She had taken many homeopathic remedies that had relieved her symptoms from time to time, but whenever she began to look back on her past she sank into despair and malaise. This sound remedy lifted her spirits enough that she remained free of pain for long periods of time and could do the things she enjoyed. This woman loved playing music, which gave her brief respites from the pain. This supported the choice of prescribing the note rather than a color. Painting and sculpting are connected to the etheric body, and music is related to the astral (mental) body, as is severe pain.

THE CHAKRAS: QUALITIES, COLORS, AND SOUNDS

This section discusses the chakras, their individual qualities, and the colors and sound remedies that work with them.

The Root Chakra—Red and Middle C

The root chakra's primary quality is a sense of grounding, defined as a realistic way of engaging and connecting with the world around us. It means we are present in ourselves, aware, alert, and resonant with our surroundings. When we are grounded, we live in our bodies, not hovering over them, which we do when our spirit is disincarnate. We also tackle life's challenges in a positive, wholesome way that allows us to validate ourselves no matter what happens.

Health in this chakra assures our ability to manage life's essentials by securing what we need to sustain life, such as food and shelter, for ourselves and our family. Survival is the main issue of this chakra. It relates to how we connect to our family, community, tribe, and nation. It also relates to organizational and administrative skills. This is the chakra where we distill order out of chaos. Via this chakra, we build, we connect, we develop, and we participate in life as fully as we can.

Patience, the ability to see projects and relationships through to their natural conclusion, is also an aspect of this chakra. We persevere and do not give up. A strong sense of grounding and determination is required to stay on track and develop our patience. People who are not grounded lack patience. They are easily victimized and frustrated and give up too soon.

Another quality the root chakra provides is the ability to create a wholesome structure for our life that is both meaningful and fulfilling. This means we allow life to unfold in healthy and creative ways that we can pursue. Structuring our time and energy so that we can make the best use of our gifts and skills helps us fulfill our destiny.

Stability is an essential quality of a healthy root chakra. Constant dramas or crises only deplete and drain our vital energy. Stability and consistency help us hold the fort when everything and everyone around us is in despair or panic. Leading a stable life, which is both rhythmic and routine, keeps us stable and on course during change.

The root chakra also offers a sense of security, which is vital. If we don't feel safe, we will never settle in, settle down, or settle into ourselves. Many people have no deep sense of inner or outer security in their lives. They live with constant threat or peril, which drains away precious life energy, creating a weakened immunity system and opening the door for illness to take hold. It is essential to feel safe in one's self and in the world in general. No one should feel threatened in their own private haven, even if it's just a small room where you can be yourself and rest. A person with little or no inner security cannot thrive.

In order to ground our creativity, we need to believe that we can manifest our dreams into reality. We must learn to trust life and believe that we are here on earth to fulfill a higher purpose. The ability to manifest our dreams into reality is a very important aspect of the root chakra.

The root chakra's functionality can become impaired whenever there is uprooting or drastic change in one's life. Dysfunction can be the result of war, poverty, divorce, separation, abuse, or disease. Cultivating trust, hope, and the belief that we are meant for joy, happiness, and goodness keep the root chakra open and expanding.

▓ THE ROOTS OF DISEASE

When homeopaths describe the roots of disease, they refer to miasms, or genetic predisposition for disease, which are reflected in the root chakra. In homeopathy, five miasms are considered to be the root causes of disease: psoric, sycotic, syphilitic, cancerous, and tubercular. A person with a psoric predisposition will be overwhelmed by struggle and conflict and want to give up.

Someone with a sycotic predisposition will want to conquer their environment and will run the risk of becoming ill from excess work. Those with a syphilitic predisposition will be unusually creative and then begin to destroy themselves in their attempts at success. Those with a cancerous predisposition will design their lives so that they remain unfulfilled or unexpressed. A tubercular miasm reflects itself in restlessness and longing. (Refer to a classical homeopathy guide for a discussion on the miasms. They are too complex to discuss in this book.) Our predispositions also mean that certain types of situations will make us susceptible to particular imbalances. How we respond is governed by our miasmatic, genetic inheritance and whether these tendencies have been treated homeopathically.

The root chakra, which stores our genetic inheritance, governs the adrenal cortex and the medulla of the kidneys. When we need to draw upon our reserves of energy, we call up what the Chinese call ancestral chi, or energy, which is stored in the adrenal cortex of the kidneys.

Whenever we fall into our chronic patterns of response, which have accumulated over generations, we are activating our "roots." This can be either positive or negative. If, for instance, people find themselves victims of life, they may need to harness their strength and reserves to create a new and better life. We have the ability to transform the victim archetype to one of mother, nurturer, healer, and giver. The choice to change is always ours.

This core vitality and strength goes beneath our primary responses and gives us the ability to rebuild a structure, create better security and more stability, and patiently reestablish order in our lives. It allows us to refashion our dreams so we are able to manifest what we need and see what we desire.

The root chakra is also related to issues of family and tribe, and the attitudes that maintain their continuity. The issues of this chakra are not related to higher consciousness as much as to survival patterns that kept the family alive. We need to ask ourselves whether we still need to be in survivor mode, or whether we can ease down into life, enjoy ourselves, create a stable and centered existence, and live creatively and productively.

▦ DETERMINING COLOR AND SOUND REMEDIES FOR THE ROOT CHAKRA

The color red and the musical note middle C are remedies we would use to treat any dysfunction of this chakra. They can be given in low potency, repeated twice a day; when stability becomes apparent, then one 30C remedy can be administered. If there is real fear about survival, then use both the color and the note at the same time.

To determine whether a person needs the note or the color, ask whether this person needs the energy of grounding or needs to reflect on survival. If it is both, then give both. If they need more energy, then the color remedy would precede the sound remedy. Give the remedy that offers the primary solution, and when they stabilize, use the other remedy.

The Sacral Chakra—Orange and the Note D

The qualities of the sacral chakra, which is located two inches below the navel and two inches into the pelvis, revolve around ease, pleasure, sexuality, creativity, and abundance. They relate to the manner in which we choose to live on the physical plane, and, ultimately, how deeply and lovingly we value ourselves. These life issues reflect how we feel about ourselves, including our bodies, our pleasures, and the things we cherish. These attitudes create vitality, good health, and physical well-being, and give us a sense that we are entitled to pleasure, wealth, beauty, and abundance.

Another aspect of this chakra is focused on how we look after our physical body in terms of cleanliness, beauty, care, exercise, proper eating, rest, and time for relaxation. Physical vitality and the ability to move freely and joyfully are also governed by this center. Pleasure is an issue for most people, and it is reflected in the ways that we open ourselves to seeking joy, happiness, and creating a standard of physical well-being.

If we are plagued by guilt and feel we must suffer, and feel burned out often, then we do not have a healthy second chakra. We wind up giving away what we want or going without pleasure because we feel our duty lies in sacrifice. We then live out a martyr's archetype.

The good we are able to enjoy strengthens and fortifies this chakra. Pleasure supports life and gives us the will and the energy to do the tasks we have set for ourselves. We choose the things we want, as well as the jobs we do.

Pleasure sustains us when life is challenging, and it recharges us for our work. It stimulates expansion at every level. How we view our right to pleasure is what defines this chakra's function.

Sexuality is part of this chakra's strength and vitality. Dysfunctional or disconnected sexuality is an indication that this center is not balanced. Problems with fertility, menstruation, or reproduction, including difficult births, suggest a person has unhealthy ideas and attitudes about sexuality. Other problems, such as premature ejaculation, impotency, and low libido, also reflect an imbalanced sacral chakra.

In general, this center is universally dysfunctional, because of the way the world generally views sexuality. Sexuality is cut off from the heart and is used as a commodity throughout the world. When people's worth is measured by their material wealth and what they have, not who they are, their sexuality will be dysfunctional.

At an energetic level, people who are dependent on constantly recharging their sacral chakra energy will repeatedly grasp the external validations of sex and money as a way of reaffirming themselves. This suggests weakness and fear at their core, as well as a lack of personal identity.

This chakra becomes strong through a rhythmic, intentional life that honors a person's body, mind, and spirit. It implies balance in all things, from what we eat to the levels of physical engagement we partake in. Learning to enjoy ourselves and finding down time from demands and stress soothes our nervous systems and replenishes this chakra.

This chakra controls the sense of appetite, so eating disorders and greed are reflected here. Interestingly, this chakra also controls the body's fluid balance. In homeopathy, we look at retentive emotions as a causative factor in fluid retention. This center also governs emotions. When people swell up, it is often suppressed emotions that they are unwilling to experience that are creating the condition.

The sacral chakra also controls our sense of abundance. A person may overemphasize or underemphasize wealth and material possessions, which raises the question of how someone feels about experiencing life's goodness. One must deeply honor one's self to value one's self above any material possessions and enjoy the beauty and power of the physical world.

◼ DETERMINING COLOR AND SOUND REMEDIES FOR THE SACRAL CHAKRA

Many physical illnesses that revolve around fatigue and exhaustion respond well to homeopathic orange and the note D. These are the resonant color and sound for the sacral chakra. They regulate and stabilize the energy flowing into the physical body through this chakra, helping people regain their health and vitality.

Orange can be used whenever there is a need for more physical vitality. It energizes this chakra and is good for people who are depleted and low of energy. When orange is combined with pink, a sense of well-being is created. Pink is associated with mother love and brings order to this center. The note D stimulates vitality and joy; it can be used by itself or together with orange where there is serious dysfunction.

The Solar Plexus Chakra—Yellow and the Note E

The solar plexus chakra relates to our sense of personal worth: knowing who we are without any veils to disguise our true nature.

Self-worth, self-esteem, confidence, and personal power are all qualities that are associated with this chakra. They reflect a deep sense of personal identity. The stronger their sense of self, the more a person takes command of their life and makes healthy choices. People who make unhealthy choices in their lives and get caught in compromising situations where they become manipulated, treated badly, or abused may have issues with personal identity. When patients speak of situations in which they cannot stand up for themselves or fight for their rights, we know they need to fortify the solar plexus chakra.

An unhealthy solar plexus chakra is reflected on a physical level by problems with the gallbladder, liver, stomach, small intestine, and pancreas. Hyperacidity, ulcers, and digestive disorders all indicate that a person is blocking feelings of aggression, fear, or anxiety. They are literally swallowing their feelings and not putting a stop to abuse in their lives.

Another aspect of the solar plexus chakra is freedom of choice. This means having the awareness to know that we can choose what we want and how we want to do things. People who have given over their power to choose and allow others to make their choices have given away their power. Calling our power back from all the projections we have created is a way in which we strengthen our solar plexus chakra and ourselves. Calling our power back empowers us and makes us whole.

Cultivating the power to live out our destiny requires a sense of purpose and worth. When we buy into any form of invalidation because of our age, sex, race, or sexual preference, we are diminished. When we collude with a negative image of ourselves we give away our power.

When we forget who we are, such as in a difficult job or a challenging relationship, and we fail to speak our truth, we weaken this center. We must believe in our worth and know that we are good and loveable and that we deserve to be treated in a loving way.

Yellow and the note E can help transform the energy of the solar plexus chakra. It focuses on issues of self-worth, confidence, personal power, and freedom of choice. Yellow can energize this chakra and provide a deeper sense of power, authority, and mastery in dealing with situations. It can provide energy to the digestive system and help tonify the liver, gallbladder, stomach, and pancreas. The musical note E can be used to reflect on issues of Selfhood and ideas about power and worth. The note helps the mind form clear ideas about who we are and what we feel we are worthy of having in this life.

The Heart Chakra—Green and Pink and the Note F

The heart chakra is concerned with all aspects of love, peace, and joy. It works on two levels. One level is the heart itself and the other is the heart protector, which acts as a shield against whatever is negative and hurtful. The heart protector corresponds to the pericardium in the physical body. This shield also acts to protect the purity and innocence of the human heart from exposure to harsh or unloving experiences. The heart protector provides a safe refuge and sanctuary for the heart to reside; it sustains the core of our being from pain and abuse.

The heart protector's core energy is made from the fabric of our experiences of love, whether that is family love, personal friendship, partnerships, love of nature, love of animals, or spiritual love. For those who have experienced deep abandonment and unloved lives, energy channeled from the spirit realm often acts to shield the heart from breaking. Love doesn't always have to be personal to sustain us. Love from many sources can keep us going forward in life. What we do need to acknowledge is that this love is all from the one Source.

All experiences that contribute to love, be they personal or impersonal, strengthen the heart protector. When we experience things as heartfelt, the inner chambers of our heart, the Holy of Holies, resound in joy.

Our heart's innocence and purity make us vulnerable. It takes love to strengthen us, sustain us, and protect us in the world. But love can send us soaring to the heights or bring us down so low we ache with pain. And when the heart has been too open or too closed, emotional pathology may result.

After a heart operation, people heal quickly when they are able to cry and release blocked emotions. The tears act to release pent-up energy that has been locked in the heart for a long while. Love keeps the two-way valve of the heart open and flowing.

The heart chakra is in the center of our energy system, just as the heart is the center of the body, and love is the center of our lives, providing the core strength that keeps us moving forward in life. Love asks us to forgive those who hurt us, move forward in our own way, and discover our own path. If love is what drives us forward, it will surely come to us in return. When we allow love to be that guiding star in our life, we draw to us those experiences and people who fulfill our yearning for love.

As we mature, we find higher levels and more refined ways of expressing and experiencing love. The expression of love may acquire a very different appearance than the one to which we were accustomed in our youth. Love of the heart transcends all barriers, all situations, great distances, and even death. Love endures in the soul and leaves an indelible mark that builds up the spirit and nourishes us. The ultimate truth is that love heals.

▨ DETERMINING COLOR AND SOUND REMEDIES FOR THE HEART CHAKRA

The colors of the heart chakra are green, for peace and balance, and pink, for universal mother love. The musical note F is the sound for this center. Both these remedies can help heal a broken heart and fortify the heart center when it is challenged.

When used to soften the heart center, green and pink create calmness and tranquility and ease tension in the heart. Green has been used for cardiac edema and angina. Pink keeps the emotions around the heart soft, gentle, and loving. The musical note F allows us to think about love, how we can open the channel for love to reach us and transform our life.

The Throat Chakra—Turquoise and the Note G

The throat chakra focuses on communication and our need to be expressive and creative. It rules our ability to share our feelings and find the right words to convey our heartfelt emotions, as well as our ideas and thoughts. Our relationship to truth—both our personal truth and the higher truth of God—affects this chakra's tonicity and functionality.

This chakra governs our integrity and willpower and affects how we cultivate our personal forces of strength, flexibility, and resiliency. At a physical level, this applies to what we eat, drink, and smoke, and whether we choose to say no to what is harmful and bad for us. All substance-abuse issues pass through the narrow opening of the throat and destroy the will. The use of bad language, cursing, and gossip also weaken this center. We need to use our will to meet the difficult challenges we face in our development.

The throat is a center for truth in all regards. That applies not only to how we communicate with others, but our ability to find what is moral, right, and truthful in ourselves. In metaphysics, this center is called "the mouth of God," because it is from here that we channel our highest good. It is said that angels whisper in our ears and bring us healing and guidance. The sense of hearing is a throat chakra function.

If we cannot cultivate a strong will or we are too busy with external affairs and fail to hear our inner guidance, this chakra becomes congested and blocked. If we allow slander, negativity, or invalidation to corrode our sense of Self, we are not valuing the precious life energy we have been given or our true nature.

Right use of will is a very important aspect of the throat chakra. When we abuse alcohol or tobacco, or when we use drugs, either recreational or allopathic medicine, we weaken our will and diminish our ability to protect ourselves against what is harmful and damaging to our core. If we persist in abusing our systems, we will find it increasingly difficult to harness our will for purposeful tasks. We will give up on ourselves and the things that really mean something to us. When this chakra is balanced, there is space for feelings to be expressed and for thoughts to arise freely.

It is through the throat chakra that we are linked to a higher source of light and truth. This is the point where we channel our Higher Self. Energy enters the back of the throat center and projects onto the front of the throat. This is where communication is expressed to the world. When we commit to being truth tellers, our integrity levels soar and our throat becomes a channel for truth, clarity, and vision.

Integrity is our ability to "walk our talk." This means that we do what we say we are going to do, to the best of our ability. Vital moral impulses work through us and find direct expression in our lives—in our relationship with others, in our work, and in the things that anchor us on this earth plane. Having integrity refers to our ability to relate to the world from the place where we are whole and complete. This is reflected in the timbre of our voice, as well as in the words we speak.

Children who have been abused, people who have been taught not to speak their truth, or those who have taken many drugs over a prolonged period of time have a very weak throat chakra. It takes a strong act of will to control our negativity, express our thoughts and feelings from a place of personal power and responsibility, and ask for what we want and what we believe is ours. Proper communication skills, which allow us to say what is in our heart in an appropriate manner, help to strengthen this chakra.

DETERMINING COLOR AND SOUND REMEDIES FOR THE THROAT CHAKRA

The color associated with the throat chakra is turquoise. It helps strengthen this center and seal off energy, which tends to dissipate as a result of blocked emotions. Turquoise can be used for physical problems with the jaw, mouth, and throat. It is also excellent for people who cannot express their emotions. The musical note G opens the ears and throat and allows for clear, resonant thinking. It can help us clear the patterns of fear associated with speaking our truth. This note can expand our hearing so that we are tuned to our higher truth.

The Brow Chakra—Indigo Blue and the Note A

The brow chakra is located between the eyebrows, and in yoga it is known as the control center. It functions as an antenna, allowing us to perceive such things as safety and danger. In a normally developed brow chakra, which begins to bud in early adolescence and becomes fully functional by the time of our Saturn return at age twenty-eight, you will find such qualities as discernment, wisdom, knowledge, intuition, and imagination taking hold. When a person is endangered, especially if they had angry or volatile parents or unsupportive siblings in childhood, this chakra will develop very quickly, even prematurely, to help them see their way through crises and adapt to change. Some of the strongest clairvoyants are those who grew up in unsafe homes or countries.

The brow chakra controls many vital functions and is our conscious link to our life choices and how we function in the world. Our imagination, an aspect of the brow chakra, is used to visualize what we want in our future. It helps us see what action we need to take and how we want events to unfold. It helps us make our dreams become reality. This is the realm of imagination.

The intuitive function of the right brain allows us to know the truth about people and situations. It helps us develop wisdom from our life experiences. Wisdom is this center's chief goal. It reflects our capacity to acquire wisdom from negative experiences in our lives and distill it into a moral impulse that can be a guiding light. We can cultivate wisdom by looking at the difficult and challenging times in our lives and asking ourselves what we learned. This way, we build a treasury of wisdom out of our hardships. It is said in the Bible that wisdom is more valuable than gold.

Knowledge about how to live a happy and useful life also contributes to a well-functioning brow chakra. Knowledge helps us upgrade our lives and move to the next level of creative expression and fulfillment. Discernment is another function of this chakra. It helps us to pick and choose who and what is best for our highest good. Like wisdom, discernment comes with time and experience. It is ultimately the way we can find our truth and stay on track with our lives. Saying no to what is painful and hurtful gives us a stronger sense of self and more energy to do what we know is right for us.

The brow chakra's five qualities—imagination, intuition, discernment, knowledge, and wisdom—make it the center of control for 90 percent of our vital functions. Those who have a highly developed brow chakra are able to master their lives. A weakened solar plexus, for example, will drain energy from the brow chakra, so energy spent proving our worth stops us from using our higher creative powers in a positive way. However, by placing positive thoughts and affirming our worth in this chakra, we not only strengthen the brow chakra but all the other chakras as well.

The brow chakra is important for developing our spiritual path. By living fully in this chakra, we learn the universal truths that govern human interaction. From here, we are better able to direct our energy to a higher spiritual plane. In the realm of the brow chakra we form clear thoughts that we can act on and that will lead us to good results in the situations we face in life.

Indigo blue is the color of the brow chakra, and the musical note A is the sound remedy. This is the color and sound of universal healing; they also represent detachment and are both cooling and remote.

Indigo works on the senses, especially the eyes. It can help the emotions detach when they become overly engaged or inflamed. It is a remedy for cooling what is heated, including a fever. The note A is for developing wise and grounded thinking about one's self, or about situations that require clear and focused thought.

The Crown Chakra—Violet and the Note B

The crown chakra sits at the top of the head. It influences pituitary and pineal functioning and governs our communion with the spirit realm, which is the highest Source of consciousness. Its function is to help us live in bliss, peace, and beauty. It strongly influences our aesthetics and helps us create harmony. It also connects us to that place within ourselves where tranquility and serenity live.

When the crown chakra is impaired, we see such health problems as epilepsy, brain tumors, strokes, and disjointed mental patterns develop. Whenever there are physical problems in this area, there will be problems facing emotional issues about growth, maturity, and natural development. People with these problems often may wish to remain in an undifferentiated, amorphic state, not wanting to grow up or mature or have to take personal responsibility for themselves. They wish to remain childish, tied to their parents, particularly their mothers, and not face the responsibilities of an adult life.

Meditation helps to stabilize this area and can show a frightened mind the truth of what is real. This chakra is known as the "thousand-petalled lotus," and it governs illumination and enlightenment, the goal of all spiritual practice. The crown chakra controls spiritual truths and higher consciousness.

Issues of spiritual growth that surface are often resolved in this chakra. The more we attempt to live our own lives and fulfill what we feel to be our higher purpose, the more we may experience difficulties, invalidation, and hardship. Each test is there to affirm our strength, clarify our resolve, and create trust in a Higher Power. The road to individuation is fraught with peril, yet something within us drives us to grow, tell our truth to those who can listen, and define ourselves in this world and with the spirit realm. That is what energy in this chakra can do to support our growth and healing.

Stabilizing the crown chakra takes time; it must move slowly. Invasive therapies or harsh medication can shock and overwhelm the nervous system, which is profoundly affected by the crown chakra.

DETERMINING COLOR AND SOUND REMEDIES FOR THE CROWN CHAKRA

Violet is the color of the crown chakra; it provides stability to this center. The musical note B also can be used to stabilize crown chakra energy. They both provide peace, act as an anesthetic, and help to control pain. Violet can also promote sleep and restful awareness. The note B helps us to think about our spiritual connections and reflect on spirit working in our life.

The Alta Major Chakra—Magenta and the Note C

The alta major chakra sits a foot above the head and relates to our link with the collective unconscious. This chakra holds information about our past and present incarnations and the contractual agreements we made with our Higher Self before this incarnation. This center is undeveloped in most people and will open up in the new age as we all become more aligned with healing and protecting this planet.

This chakra is our telepathic link to the akashic records, which are the repository of all knowledge and activity from all time. The alta major chakra acts as a communication link with the spirit realm, and when it is in balance we know and love ourselves, and the world around us, at a deep and profound level. The more we love who we are, the more we accept our oneness with the Creator and the more we have clear intentionality about our role in making our world whole, beautiful, and complete.

▪ DETERMINING COLOR AND SOUND REMEDIES FOR THE ALTA MAJOR CHAKRA

The color of the alta major chakra is magenta, which incorporates the properties of red, green, and violet. The musical note is high C. This color and sound give us spiritual understanding and a sense of creative purpose in our lives. They allow us to be repositories of the collective unconscious and to find guidance from higher spiritual realms.

Magenta provides wisdom and insight into a situation and helps us look at the bigger picture. High C helps us to think universally, focusing our awareness on a larger horizon than we have normally been used to.

CHAPTER FOUR

The Color and Sound Remedies and Their Qualities

The qualities of the color and sound remedies can lead you to discover which remedy would work best for you or your client. We use the qualities to understand the deeper nature of our problems, and if we are lacking in one particular quality we have the opportunity to cultivate that in our life. We can use these qualities as benchmarks for our development and growth.

RED AND THE NOTE MIDDLE C

Red and the note middle C are the sound and color of the root chakra, which deals with survival, administration, organization, structure, and security. This center focuses on the emotional qualities of patience, stability, structure, security, and the ability to make our dreams come true. If a person is able to live sufficiently from this center, they are ready to create the next level of their life, a level that relates to pleasure, sexuality, financial abundance, and well-being.

Red

Red is the color of life. It flows through our bodies. It is found in all forms of nature, from the red clay of the earth to the garish feathers of a desert cardinal flying from cactus to cactus. We value red for its vibrancy; we love it as a metaphor for courage, vitality, and even danger.

Red has the slowest vibration and most dense energy field of any color. It also has the longest wavelength and the lowest energy level of all colors. It is a heavy color with no respite from engagement. Red forces us to notice it, whatever its form may take. When we see red, we are pulled into it and connected with it, whether we want to be or not.

We notice red; it is the first color the human eye will see in a series of colors. It is used to alert the senses and to convey messages of caution. It is believed that very early man could see only red, yellow, and black—the colors of warning. As we have evolved, our ability to identify color has developed, but red remains the primary color that the eye distinguishes from all others.

Red relates to the planet Saturn and governs our physical and material existence. It is the first color to intrude on the senses when one has been in a darkened space. It is believed that, of all colors, babies see red first because it is the color that has surrounded them for many months.

Red carries the greatest emotional impact of any color. It is the color of passion, lust, and violence. It pulls us in and heats us up. It warms our feelings. It is impossible to be impassive and remote in its field. Long exposure to red is said to quicken the heart rate, cause adrenaline to be released into the bloodstream, and give a sense of warmth. Red stimulates our senses, and people sitting under red light for more than a few minutes report a heavy, leaden feeling, irritation and anger, and a quickening of the pulse.

When things are painted red, they appear nearer than they truly are. Red has the effect of making spaces appear small and congested. It is a color that demands attention and says, "*Here I am. Look at me; see me.*" Its conspicuous power makes it the obvious color to wear when giving commands. It is used in military uniforms because it is believed to charge the blood and lend courage. This color is linked to combat, aggression, and a martial spirit.

Color has long been used in medical diagnoses, and red suggests inflammation and a quality of disorganized blood, seen especially on people's faces when they are excited or frightened. Red is also associated with body heat. In China the word for *blood* translates as "blood red." The first association with this color is that of our own blood.

Red feeds and nourishes the blood. It is associated with the heart and is used in healing to enhance circulation. It is also associated with the physical, carnal aspects of life. Too much red has been known to raise blood pressure and create irritability and anger. We have an expression in English that when we are angry "we see red." This could be the result of elevated blood pressure, which inflames the blood vessels in the eye and actually creates an optical vision of red.

The bond between earth, life, and red is found in every culture on our planet. Rituals involving blood, for both men and women, are found in all tribal societies. Tribesmen in Kenya drink the blood of their cattle for nourishment and strength. They honor red as the essence of life. They also wear red-dyed robes to honor life. Graves found in prehistoric sites in East Africa were painted with red ochre. The poet William Butler Yeats said that red was the color of magic in every country and has been so since the very earliest times. Red is synonymous with life.

Esoterically, red represents the final stage in alchemy before turning base lead into gold. It had great import for the old alchemists, who were the precursors to homeopaths. Anger is often thought to be the final step before enlightenment, with alchemy corresponding to the inner stages of awareness.

Red is associated with iron and can be given whenever the blood is lacking that mineral. It is indicated for anemia or any immunodeficiency disease, whether it is given with colored lights or in homeopathic potency. Red works well when people need to be earthed, or grounded, to bring them out of their mind and into their body and feelings.

When people are recovering from illness or when they have been uprooted from their ordinary life through loss, shock, or trauma, this color helps them regain their footing, becoming grounded. Red stimulates a person's sense of their right to existence. It is also indicated whenever healthy boundaries have been violated. It enhances our sense of place and promotes passions that we need in order to choose a meaningful and fulfilled life. Red suggests independence and freedom.

People who need red are infirm and weak, low in their life force, or too involved with the spirit realm and not "on the ground." It is a color with great vital energy. It can be used homeopathically for people who have inflammations on the physical level or deep emotional suppression that keeps them disconnected from their reality.

Too much red can create hemorrhage and an overflow of feeling, and it is to be used cautiously. It is suggested that a medium potency be given and the patient be observed over a period of three to four days before repeating the remedy.

When we use homeopathic remedies such as ferrum, or cinnabaris, which is mercurius sulphate, we would not use red as a support remedy, as these remedies contain large quantities of this color. Mercurius sulphate is a red mineral that has all the characteristics of a person with an abundance of red in their energy field. Its picture contains violence and manipulation and reflects an emotional person who is suspicious and seeks to hold onto power, in other words, a person who is very red by nature.

Mercurius sulphate creates inflammation of the bones, burning pains, and swollen glands, which can inflame and indurate. Mercurius sulphate patients fear murder and being murdered, poverty, dirt, and ugliness. This reflects a deeply dysfunctional root chakra, having an excess of red energy congested and blocked in this chakra.

It would be best to use one of the higher colors to help decongest the red energy in this patient's chakra. It is evident with mercurius sulphate that, at a certain level, there is also an impaired crown chakra where spirituality is not being nurtured and the moral impulses are not connected with a higher spiritual consciousness.

Red can also be combined with plant remedies, especially those that survive in winter and have a healing effect on the vital force, such as *Helleborus, Bryonia,* and *Arnica.* These remedies possess a high vital force that is capable of restoring vitality in those who are weak or prostrated. Carbo vegetalis and Carbo animalis also possess red energy and can be used in conjunction with red to awaken, enliven, and restore low vitality.

Red should not be given to someone who is unable to express their rage or anger. It will stimulate these emotional forces they have blocked or deeply suppressed and may create an explosive reaction. For example, in the original provings, red 30C stimulated one woman's emotions right before her menstrual period to the point that she tried to stab her husband with a fork. Her emotions ran high and she had no filter to control herself. Red needs to be given with caution to someone with emotional issues, certainly not above a 12C potency and not repeated frequently. The patient should be warned that they could become very irritable.

Homeopathic red can be used very successfully to stimulate the birthing process and gently help bring new life into the world. It stimulates the cervix to dilation. Conversely, it should not be given to anyone who is terminally ill and ready to pass over. They would need green for peace or violet for spirituality.

Wherever people are slow to react to life, need grounding, or lack strength, red is the color to consider. It can be given to sick people in very low potency to help their vitality if they are infirm and their vital forces are slow to reactivate. However, in treating the elderly, do consider using magenta, as it is a more appropriate remedy.

The Note Middle C

When the note middle C was being proved as a remedy by four women at the same time in the same room, they all experienced a feeling of stony heaviness, solidity, and a lack of mentality. These were intelligent and active women who, after taking the remedy, became slow and lethargic and felt like they had "turned to stone." They had trouble thinking and sat very still for long periods of time without speaking or connecting with one another. The women reported feeling strong, present, and unyielding. One woman said she felt she had lost her "mind" because she had no thoughts.

This is the homeopathic signature of the middle C sound remedy, and it suggests widespread use for people who are slow to move, slow to think, and slow to react. It would be an excellent remedy for those who have problems recovering from chronic illness or who have suffered a head injury and are slow to regain their clarity and get "up to speed" in their life. This may prove to be an excellent remedy for head injuries.

Middle C is also useful for treating Alzheimer's disease, where the mental functions deteriorate quickly and the ability to think clearly slows down. It can be used when memory is impaired, mental energy is low or lacking, or when people need to ground their mental processes, because it relates to rhythm, organization, rules, and regulations.

This remedy, as with all sound remedies, works on the astral forces, which control thinking, aversions, and desires. It can be used to help people who fail to think about their lives and need more mental stimulation. Middle C helps to focus thinking on survival issues since it corresponds to the root chakra.

This musical note has helped people who felt disconnected from their homes and families. It works to reestablish the links between Self and home, Self and community, Self and country, Self and the earth. Whenever there has been an interruption in the cycles and rhythms of one's life, this remedy helps to reestablish those basic rhythmic patterns of existence within ordinary life. This sound remedy can be used after a divorce, separation, house move, or any other fundamental change in one's life.

Middle C helps a person focus their mind on the essentials of life, who and what are important to their well-being, and how grateful they are for life. This sound remedy is made in only one potency, 5X, and can be given two or three times daily for a few days. It supports mental healing, gratitude, and self-acceptance.

Red and Middle C Uses

Red and middle C can be used together or separately for the following conditions.

▓ PHYSICAL PROBLEMS

Red and middle C can help people with poor circulation; constipation; piles, rectal and urinary troubles; problems with the feet, knees, or legs; childbirth; slow onset of labor; anemia; weakness; slow recuperative ability; immunodeficiency diseases, HIV, and AIDS; or dementia.

Contraindications: Red and middle C should not be given to people with high blood pressure or who are violent and aggressive by nature. Keep the potency of red under 12C initially to see how people respond. When you feel that their vital force is able to handle 30C, move to the next potency. Watch for changes before repeating and do not repeat this color too often. Move to middle C if there is irritation with red. Do not give these remedies at night. You can use red and middle C together when someone is really deeply traumatized and disconnected. Red and middle C would have the effect of bringing their consciousness back into their body and making them very present.

■ EMOTIONAL ISSUES

Red and middle C address issues of lack of grounding and feelings of disconnection, not belonging to home, family, community, or the planet. These remedies work for people who are spaced out. It is suited when there are feelings of detachment with little or no affect or emotional expression, or a lack of emotional awareness.

These remedies can be used for unstable people who have no structure to their life, who are unable to patiently await their goodness to unfold, who have trouble settling in a place, or who are unable to see a horizon in their life. Red and middle C can be used for deep depression and anxiety about survival. It is good for suicidal tendencies and long-term unhappiness.

Contraindications: Do not give red or middle C to people with a history of violence. Do not give these remedies at night.

■ MENTAL ISSUES

Red and middle C are good for people who are absorbed in spiritual practices and do not think about the practical realities of life, people who are very detached and live in another sphere of reality, dreamers, and indolent people who are unable to work or support themselves.

Contraindications: Do not give red or middle C often to people who suppress rage and channel their feelings into rationality. Do not give these remedies at night.

Red and middle C can be used for people who are locked into giving their spiritual energy to others, who do not feel they have a right to their own life, who are enslaved and unable to freely live their lives, and who need spiritual courage to make the next move in their life. At this level, red and middle C give courage and help people find the inner resources to break destructive and unwholesome patterns.

These remedies also can be used for abandoned babies, those put up for adoption, and adults who were orphaned at a young age. These remedies help all those who were abused and lost their connection to their right to their own life.

Red and Middle C Essence

The quintessential quality of red and middle C is imploded, congested, or compacted energy—energy turned in on itself, not connected with an external presence or reality. Red is hot. Middle C is the base note. These remedies provide energy that is contracted and full of vitality, but potentially explosive. The energy is intense, dense, and slow moving.

Red provides heat, shelter, strength, and nourishment. Middle C gives stability and steadiness in the face of change. It forces people to think about themselves and their situation. These remedies relate to the mother archetype and the life force found in our blood. People who comprise this archetype ask to be contained, held in, or held back. For example, someone with the victim archetype has little or no stability, and red and middle C can act as stabilizers. They help ground, anchor, and connect.

Homeopathic Remedies Related to Red and Middle C

All the ferrums contain the energy of red and the vibration of middle C. They are also associated with mercury and fluorine, which contain this base vibration. Plant remedies that have this energy are *Berberis*, *Arnica*, Carbo vegetalis, Carbo animalis, belladonna, and nux vomica. Both *Lachesis* and *Naja* (snake remedies used for rebalancing the energy system), spider poisons, and scorpion all reflect root chakra energy and life issues.

Caution: Red and middle C are used in cases where a person's physical vitality is weakened. These remedies can provoke rage and anger if these emotions have been deeply suppressed. They can bring out violence and antisocial behavior in people who are already too hot emotionally. Use them with care. If necessary, use a higher color, such as indigo or violet, as an antidote.

Red and Middle C Cases

Here are cases that demonstrate how these remedies have been used therapeutically.

▦ CASE ONE: HOMEOPATHIC RED

A man, age thirty-seven, had suffered from Epstein-Barr virus for three years and was so weak he could not work and had to go on welfare. He was better out of doors and in the country, and he craved fresh air. He developed a strong desire (passion) for being out on the land. He was treated with several homeopathic remedies for over a year, which helped him regain his energy. When he was given red 12C three times daily for a month, his energy levels soared. He was able to start a new work project that allowed him to work from his home on his own hours and thus earn a living. He continued to have frequent relapses of Epstein-Barr, but he recovererd quickly each time he took another treatment. Eventually, over a few years, he fully regained his energy with the use of red. He began on red 6X, repeated three times daily, moved up to the red 12C three times daily for a month, and eventually proceeded to 12C twice a day. After many months, he began taking one dose of 30C daily, and finally he took one single dose of 30C as needed every few months.

▥ CASE TWO: HOMEOPATHIC MIDDLE C

A woman, age fifty-seven, who worked long shifts as a nurse and looked after an aging mother at the same time, did well on middle C given as a single dose. Within days of taking the remedy, she changed her workload and got help for her mother. She realized that she was a slave to her fixed ideas about helping others. Her healing came in recognizing that she believed she had a duty to sacrifice her life for others. This remedy helped her regain a belief in her right to her own life. She immediately began to question herself about what she was doing with her life and implemented changes that took her needs into account. She repeated the remedy whenever she fell back into her old patterns.

▥ CASE THREE: HOMEOPATHIC RED

A woman, approximately fifty years old, had involuntary stools each time she urinated. She had tried several remedies, which did not assuage her problem, and she was considering surgery. Taking one dose of red 30C a week alleviated all of her distressing symptoms.

A thirty-seven-year-old woman with chronic anemia used middle C to fortify her blood and strengthen her awareness. She was very courageous and lived a life rich with integrity and service to others. Middle C helped her to consciously choose her spiritual path and to keep her life force anchored in her body. She stopped suffering from fatigue and exhaustion in her work and became clear about how she could best serve others and meet her own needs as well. The sound remedy helped her think clearly about what she wanted to do with her life and how she could implement changes that worked on her behalf. She took the remedy three times daily for several weeks until her thinking patterns began to shift.

ORANGE AND THE NOTE D

The second chakra, known as the sacral chakra, is the center of joy, creativity, and pleasure. It governs ease, movement, pleasure, sensuality and sexuality, well-being, and abundance. It is ruled by the archetype of the empress/emperor, who lives abundantly in the material world and enjoys the good things of life. This archetype is a metaphor for pleasure, as are orange and the note D.

The sacral chakra and its corresponding archetypes are associated with people who have a healthy appetite for life. Orange and the note D both govern a person's appetite, as the advertising industry so clearly knows. Observe the way cheap junk food advertisements are printed in orange. They appeal to the appetite on a subliminal level. Conversely, too much orange or vibration of the note D in a person's system reveals a sign of greed, an indication that the person feels they are not enough and need to compensate for those feelings. This manifests at a psychological level as wanting or needing more. This may manifest as desiring more food, more experience, more sex, or more money, but all reflect a belief that what they have in their life is not enough.

The sacral chakra controls the water element of the body and is essential in regulating the flow of our emotions. A deficiency of orange or D in the human energy system is also linked with allergies; this means that the energetic sheaths that protect us from invasive assault are weak and need fortifying. We have also found in the provings that the craving for chocolate relates to emotional suppression and a deep longing for love. This has been transformed when the homeopathic orange or note D remedy has been given.

Patients get a tremendous sense of joy and well-being from these color and sound remedies. One prover said she laughed all day and found herself giggling for no apparent reason. This is why it has been used so successfully for depressed and suicidal patients. The two remedies have been used to treat low spirits and have been successful in lifting the energy of chronically depressed patients.

Orange and the note D provide us with a vibration that stimulates our sense of joy and enlivens our physical vitality. They restore a sense of humor. These remedies also help people who are deficient in sexual energy to regain a sense of pleasure, nourishing and stimulating the sexual organs and getting the hormones flowing again. This serves both people who have depleted their sexual center from overuse or who have not had any sexual contact for a long period of time. It is also useful when people have negative attitudes that inhibit their sexual function, or lack a sense of ease and joy in relation to their bodies. These remedies relate directly to a sense of pleasure. They can be given as a tonic when vitality is low, especially after an illness. They should never be given at night because the energy of the remedies will keep people from relaxing into sleep.

These two remedies can be used to stimulate lazy bowels and to help relieve slow onset of the menses. They can be recommended for girls with irregular periods, such as homeopathic pulsatilla types or calcium carbonicum constitutionals. However, they are not suggested for women who have a tendency to flood during menstruation.

Since orange and D both govern the water element in the body, they can be used as active diuretics to stimulate urination and ease PMS. Provers repeatedly mentioned frequent urination and a need to cry over things that disturbed them when taking the remedy. Water imbalance is directly related to suppressed emotions, and orange and D seem to activate the body's ability to release fluid and reanimate feelings. It is much gentler than the violent emotions released from using red.

Orange and D stimulate physical energy. They can also be considered for infertility if a couple is having trouble conceiving. These remedies, along with good constitutional treatment, can stimulate fertility and help bring on pregnancy. They are life-enhancing and life-promoting. It is suggested that they be used around the time of ovulation and given approximately five times daily for five days.

These remedies can cause emotional upsets and displays of anger if used too frequently, especially by people whose tempers run high and who anger quickly. In the provings, people enjoyed being social more than usual and liked to be close to one another. In the proving of D, the people taking the remedy all wanted to stay together and eat together, and they actually all ordered orange food in a restaurant. They were more friendly than usual while taking the remedy. A high sociability factor fits closely with this chakra and orange and D can help shy people overcome their timidity.

Orange

Orange, in its various shades of coral, apricot, sienna, and umber, is the color for people who are enthusiastic about life and are eager to participate and engage with others. It is the color of vitality, and, in shades of pale orange and apricot, it represents the sensual side of our nature and addresses our love of pleasure. On the whole, it is a warm, positive, and vibrant color that lifts flagging energy and gives a bright, affirmative quality to those who wear it or decorate with it.

Orange has only one negative association; it can represent excess or indulgence, and people sometimes need the higher colors to balance lusty appetites. Orange combined with turquoise or pale blue can create a spiritual balance. Many churches throughout the world combine orange, or terra-cotta, and blue in their buildings. This signifies heaven and earth. It is a mixture of the physical and the spiritual. This is also seen in jewelry from the Native Americans and Tibetans, who often mix turquoise and carnelian or coral.

Psychologically, orange behaves like yellow, sharing depth, intensity, and brightness as an aspect of its nature. Orange is cheerful, expansive, rich in energy and vibrancy, and extroverted.

This suggests that a person who has the heat and warmth of orange about them would also be confident, be powerful, and have an abundant sense of self-worth and self-esteem.

In Europe, there were no words for orange until the Middle Ages, when the fruit of the same name arrived from Arabia. Previously, things that were orange were perceived as an aspect of red. For instance, red hair, red clay, and even fire, which is distinctly orange, were called red. The color is also associated with the metals of copper, brass, and bronze. They all have an orange tint to them. In ancient alchemy, tin was the metal that corresponded with the sacral chakra. It is the metal linked with orange.

Orange energy is found in amber, citrine, quartz, and topaz, which is a Sanskrit word for fire. Many birds and mammals have orange coloring. It is also a color that is suggestive of food, and many highly nutritious foods are orange. One of the provers felt like redecorating her kitchen while taking the orange color remedy. She wanted to paint her walls orange. Color analysts know that decorators who use orange have a high success rate, mostly because it makes a space feel warm and inviting.

The color stands for fecundity and, in the Middle Ages, it had a sexual connotation. In an earlier bridal custom, brides were adorned with orange blossoms, which symbolized fertility. In fashion, orange is in constant demand and found in different shades and hues all year long because it addresses our sensuality.

When orange is mixed with pink in the homeopathic color remedies, it opens people up to a sense of fun and enjoyment. Some homeopathic nitric acid or nitrogen patients, who had difficulty allowing themselves to feel joy, benefited from using orange and pink in combination. When faced with a long and boring task, pink 3X and orange 12C in combination help to bring a sense of pleasure back into a person's life. Again, do not give these remedies at night, as they cause sleep disturbances.

The Note D

The musical note D brings joy and laughter as a tonic for overly serious people. In the provings, an entire group of near strangers started laughing out loud and enjoyed one another in a moment of ease and delight immediately upon taking the remedy. This remedy is used to stimulate sweetness and joy in a person bereft of these qualities who may have suffered too long.

The note D engenders laughter and happiness and can be used for people who are joyless, uncomfortable in social situations, or are too strict in allowing themselves pleasure. It can be used to help people reflect on the nature of pleasure in their lives and how they want that to manifest. It can aid people who have experienced loss or separation. It supports people when times are challenging and their energy is low. It can be used as a tonic for the astral forces when illness has required prolonged rest and recuperation.

Orange and D Uses

Here are ways orange and D can be use therapeutically for healing.

PHYSICAL PROBLEMS

Consider orange and/or D for bowel problems, infertility, menstrual period irregularity, slow onset of menstruation, anorexia, or appetite disorders, including people who have little or no appetite or have food cravings for chocolate and sweets. These remedies are good for people who have postviral conditions, including difficulty recovering their natural vitality after their illness. They are good for postoperative recovery and after dentistry, emotional shock, or trauma. Orange and D are excellent for menopause, myalgic encephalomyelitis (ME, also known as chronic fatigue syndrome), multiple sclerosis (MS), and other autoimmune diseases, such as HIV and AIDS.

Contraindications: Orange and D should not be given to people who have excessive anger or rage. Nor do they suit someone with an abundance of energy, as the person may become overstimulated and restless. These remedies should not be given at night.

▧ EMOTIONAL ISSUES

Orange and D suit people who are depressive or feeling low emotionally. They have been used successfully along with Saccharine officianalis in 30C potency to help people who feel suicidal. They have been used on their own for depression and emotional "funk" for people whose feelings were blocked at a subconscious level and needed releasing. Both remedies also bring people into the present if they tend to feel spacey, allowing them to refocus their awareness into their physical body.

The note D, because it works on the astral, or mental, plane, helps people think positively about the things they enjoy and like doing. It helps people connect with their sexuality and desire for pleasure and their right to abundance. Orange is known as the "laughing color," as the provers found themselves happy and laughing much more than usual. Interestingly enough, everyone wanted "more." Therefore, it could be considered a remedy for overindulgence, binge eating, and excess.

During the provings, people cried more while on these remedies, releasing pent-up feelings that had been dormant. All the provers said that their sense of well-being was increased while on orange and the note D.

Contraindications: Neither orange nor D should be used with hyperactive people, nor should they be used at night.

MENTAL AND SPIRITUAL ISSUES

Orange and D are suited for anyone lacking a sense of their own well-being. These two remedies offer people who have a negative attitude about their bodies and sexuality an opportunity to open up and develop a healthy degree of self-acceptance. They bring an awareness of the nature of pleasure and stimulate an appetite for the good things in life. They increase interest in sexuality and abundance. D can nourish creativity, playfulness, and fun, and it helps people find what is simple and delightful in life.

Contraindications: Orange should not be given to people who are persistently restless or anxious, nor should it be used at night. D should be used only during daytime.

Orange and D Essence

The essence of both orange and D as homeopathic color and sound remedies is a joyful, very physical state of being that nurtures life and its more pleasurable aspects. This essence resonates with joy, health, and vitality, and it can bring people who are locked up with excessive overintellectualization into the present. These remedies help people to feel their emotions if they are cut off from their feelings. They can also help release negativity and feelings of despair.

Homeopathic Remedies Related to Orange and D

Homeopathic remedies such as *Berberis vulgaris, Calendula, Bellis perennis, Rhus tox,* and *Ruta graveolens* fit the sacral chakra's vibration. They also correspond to D and orange. The homeopathic mineral remedies that correspond to orange are beryllium, selenium, titanium, and tungsten. These remedies give strength and vitality. People who are Natrum types also have an affinity for orange because they retain fluid and emotions. Natrum types are generally closed emotionally and very duty-bound. They benefit from doses of D because it helps them reflect on the possibilities of pleasure in their lives. People living in Natrum climates, such as Northern Europe and Britain, where the weather is cold and damp, would feel revitalized with occasional doses of orange and D.

Orange and D Cases

Here are cases that describe ways of using orange and D in healing.

CASE ONE: HOMEOPATHIC ORANGE

A young man who suffered with chronic fatigue syndrome was prescribed orange 12C to take three times daily, along with his homeopathic constitutional remedy. Within a few weeks, he had recovered his strength and stability to the point where he could fully participate in his previous activities. Whenever he flagged and needed energy, he repeated the remedy. He found both the energy he wanted and the healing he needed for his depleted nervous system. Orange is a tonic for chronic disease states, where people are diminished and compromised.

CASE TWO: HOMEOPATHIC D

A young woman, age thirty-five, suffering from reoccurring back pains, with chronic spasms, fatigue, and irritability was given the note D three times daily for several weeks. Taking this sound remedy along with a homeopathic constitutional treatment, she managed to assuage her pain and cultivate a positive and more self-affirming attitude. She did very well on this remedy. She continued to repeat it whenever she became tired or suffered from back pain, and it took away her discomfort. It relaxed her and made her turn her thoughts to things she enjoyed. After taking the remedy, she played the flute for pleasure. During these times, she was completely pain free.

CASE THREE: HOMEOPATHIC ORANGE

The orange color remedy served a woman with chronically low energy. She was never diagnosed with any particular syndrome, but she was always tired and low-spirited, never finding the energy she needed to do her tasks. After a single dose of orange 30C, she had more vitality and higher spirits. She was advised to call whenever her energy flagged, but was never heard from after her first follow-up, when she said she felt wonderful and was very happy for the first time in a while.

CASE FOUR: HOMEOPATHIC D

Homeopathic D was given to a man with high stress levels who was nervous, fretful, and unhappy. Shortly after taking the remedy twice daily for two days, he reported feeling lighter, less involved with his case load, and more able to enjoy himself. He took time off from demands of work and reported enjoying his family more.

He said he felt more balanced, able to manage both his responsibilities and his pleasures.

YELLOW AND THE NOTE E

Yellow is the brightest of all colors in the visible spectrum, and it contains more light than any other color. The musical note E and yellow relate to the solar plexus chakra. They both convey power and presence, a sense of worth, and healthy self-esteem. Both are associated with the sun and with the metal gold.

Yellow is a warm color that gives off heat, though it is less intense than orange or red. Yellow and E can lift the spirits and give people a sense of ease and lightness; they can also help people connect to their power, deepen their sense of freedom, and acknowledge their self-worth. Most people respond to the color and the note, which represent hope and faith in the future, in a positive manner.

At a deep level, yellow and the note E affect our sense of self-worth. This is reflected in our confidence levels and the ways in which we value ourselves in relation with others. Our self-esteem and personal power show that we know who we are and what we want from life. These qualities are best represented in the warrior archetype. The dysfunctional archetype represented here is the servant, who has a diminished sense of self and weakened levels of personal power.

The association of yellow and E with the solar plexus chakra implies that a person has a healthy ego. However, too much of either the note or the color leads to an overly developed ego, and too little suggests taking a cowardly approach to challenges, or, as the slang implies, this person is a "yellow belly." From time to time, a person may need a hero's dose of courage. Yellow and E can stimulate the energy in this chakra for that. They also help balance the chakra if someone is overly inflated. Yellow given with its complement color violet works well for high levels of inflation.

Yellow lights up a drab and dull environment. It can bring a sense of radiance to clothing or a dull wardrobe. Too much yellow or too much emphasis on the note E suggests that a person is overly concerned with power and self-aggrandizement. New shades of yellow, recently developed by the automobile manufacturer BMW, suggest power and prowess on the road. They have names like Dakar Yellow (named for a challenging car race) and are reminiscent of endurance rallies.

Yellow symbolizes enlightenment because it is the color that contains the most light. The note E represents the intellect, the brighter part of the mind. Yellow has the highest reflectivity of all colors and appears to radiate outward, or to advance. The note E exemplifies the faith and hope of warmth and love, which is emotional light.

In the provings, people with fears and anxieties had an affinity for yellow and E, which helped them get over periods of doubt and worry. These remedies helped end a bout of gallbladder colic in one prover who had suffered for several days with distressing symptoms before taking the remedy. Yellow generally strengthens people who have low self-esteem and helps others make clear and intelligent choices. All provers said this remedy made them feel better about themselves and boosted their confidence. One prover became pregnant while on yellow.

Yellow

Yellow is a primary color and cannot be made by mixing other colors. For instance, orange is a combination of yellow and red; green is a combination of yellow and blue. Yellow is more closely associated with light and bright spirits than any other color.

Yellow is a diffuse and radiant energy, and if a person is not well centered, it can create an aura of confusion and make it hard to locate boundaries. Because there is so much light within this color, it can cause people to become disoriented and "spaced out," not knowing where their center is. In terms of personal development, yellow is associated with a lack of personal identity.

This color is also connected with our personal power and prowess. Through its association with gold, it relates to qualities of worth and value. It is the color of the solar plexus chakra, which represents our sense of self-worth, self-esteem, confidence, personal power, and freedom of choice.

Many body secretions are yellow and so are many foods and vitamins that we ingest. This suggests the presence of sulphur, which is a homeopathic remedy that works on the egoic forces in our personality. Sulphur is bright yellow in color.

Yellow directly affects our digestion and stimulates the stomach, pancreas, liver, and gallbladder. Too much yellow in a person's system produces jaundice or an oversecretion of bilirubin, which signifies a weakened gallbladder and liver. Too little yellow in a person's system suggests that they are not assimilating nutrients properly, and they may have problems with absorption.

Yellow is associated with the fire element required for proper absorption of nutrients. Like the sun, the color yellow implies that, when we are well in ourselves, we too shine and our systems function well. Physically and psychologically, the ability to digest our nutrients and our life experiences defines our state of health.

In food, this energy level signals the presence of vitamin A and C. Different shades of yellow evoke either the astringency of lemons and citrus or the richness of butter and cheese. In nature, yellow is caused by carotenoids and sometimes by the presence of melanin.

In the animal world, yellow is a color of warning. It is seen in tropical fish, insects, and exotic poisonous frogs. The subdued yellow of the big cats acts as a perfect camouflage for hiding in the tall, parched grasses of the bush. Such animals, like the lion and tiger, who display yellow coats, often have great presence and power.

In the early Sung dynasty in China, yellow was adapted as the imperial color, to be worn only by the emperor, his retinue, or someone wearing imperial regalia. Buddhist monks wear yellow as a sign of humility and renunciation. It is a color seen more in the Orient than in the West. In the West, yellow has been used to describe cowardice among soldiers.

The Note E

The note E has been used to support clear and intentional thinking when people need to make wholesome choices for their lives. It fosters a sense of Selfhood, which may have been arrested or never developed. If a sense of Self is weak, then the organs of digestion will also be weak. The note E stimulates both the digestive process and the mental process of claiming one's power, and strengthening a sense of personal identity. The musical note E helped a woman who lacked confidence speak out about the things she had held bottled inside her for a long while. It gave her clarity of mind, focus, and ease in expressing her intellectual ideas.

Yellow and E Uses

Here are some cases that describe the use of yellow and E.

■ PHYSICAL PROBLEMS

Yellow and E relate to the digestive organs and are most suited for treating stomach, liver, gallbladder, and pancreas symptoms. These remedies help to decongest blocked energy in the abdomen and are considered for any type of gastric colic. They can be helpful with diabetes, stomach disease, hepatitis A and B, and cancer of the liver or other digestive organs. They have been known to work on gallbladder colic, eliminating pain and congestion. They can be excellent remedies for assimilation problems, such as celiac disease, and can be used concurrently with other remedies that further enhance assimilation.

Both yellow and the note E stimulate the right eye and improve eyesight. According to Chinese theory, the eyes are controlled by the liver. Provers noted improved vision and were able to read without glasses when on these remedies.

When the vital force is low, yellow and E help unblock congestion and shift energy. They are extremely useful for colds and weakened lungs because they act as an astringent and work to unblock and decongest the bowels.

When there is an excess of yellow in the system, it is wise to use the complementary colors of purple and violet, or the note high C. When new babies are born with weakened livers and an excess of bilirubin in the blood, they are jaundiced. The standard treatment in hospitals is to place these babies under ultraviolet light for a few hours every day to break up the congestion in the blood. Homeopathic violet and high C can also help with this.

Contraindications: Yellow and the note E should be used as an astringent or a decongestant. They should be used in daytime only, as they can cause sleep disturbances.

▨ EMOTIONAL ISSUES

Yellow and the note E can be used for issues of confidence, lack of a sense of worth, low self-esteem, or a shaky sense of personal identity. It is particularly well suited to people who give their energy and life force over to others too easily and are too open in their solar plexus chakra. These remedies strengthen the ego and help people develop their individuality. Where there is emotional weakness or vulnerability, they stimulate confidence and encourage personal empowerment.

Contraindications: People with an excessively developed ego should not use yellow and E, unless they balance it with homeopathic violet or high C, as they can increase their sense of self-importance. They should not be used at night.

▨ MENTAL AND SPIRITUAL ISSUES

Yellow and E represent gut level intellect. These remedies stimulate the mind to help it become clear and focused. They help to transfer "gut knowing," which comes from the solar plexus chakra, to a higher mental level. They can be used to help increase memory and thinking ability, and they provide a rich potential for clarity and effectiveness. These two remedies help a person identify where they are weak and how they can grow in wisdom and maturity. They support empowerment, responsibility, and accountability, and in that way, promote moral impulses.

Contraindications: Too much yellow or E can cause a dissociated feeling from an overexpansion of the mind. Use during the daylight hours.

Yellow and E Essence

The essence of yellow and the note E is their remarkable brightness and diffusion of energy. The color is radiant and the sound clear. They help people shine on an inner plane and claim their power and worth. The energy resembles gold on the material plane and, therefore, relates to earthly power and worth. On the spiritual plane, the energy represents lightness of mind, a willingness to transcend the limited ego, and an opening to the power of a higher plane. Yellow and E help people feel good about themselves and let their inner light shine.

Homeopathic Remedies Related to Yellow and E

Many homeopathic remedies that work on the issues of ego identification relate to yellow and E. They correspond to silica, arsenicosum album, sulphur, fluoride, antimony, cadmium, oxygen, nitrogen, as well as *Helioanthus, Bellis perennis, Berberis,* and broom. Many of the plant remedies are yellow and work on digestion, assimilation, or repairing the body's digestive organs. Other deep-acting plant remedies, such as *Lycopodium* and *Chelidonium,* work to create a stronger ego function and address liver and gallbladder problems.

Yellow and E Cases

Here are cases that describe the use of yellow and E in healing.

CASE ONE: HOMEOPATHIC YELLOW

Homeopathic yellow was prescribed for a businessman whose authority was being challenged in important meetings. He reported that the remedy helped; each time he took it, he felt more confident, able to stand up for himself, and less stressed afterward. He continued to take it whenever he needed extra strength in facing controversial issues and difficult people. It strengthened his egoic forces.

CASE TWO: HOMEOPATHIC E

A homeopathic student who suffered from lack of inner resolution and determination took homeopathic E. After taking a single dose of the remedy, she was clearer, better able to focus her mind, and able to concentrate on her studies. It also helped her clarify her personal issues so she could heal them. She took it as needed throughout her studies.

CASE THREE: HOMEOPATHIC YELLOW

Homeopathic yellow was prescribed in a 6X potency, along with a low-potency homeopathic remedy, for a woman suffering from gallbladder dysfunction. Afterward, she was better able to digest her food, assimilate it, and pass it out. She repeated the remedy twice a day after eating and found that it supported her digestion, without any acid reflux. She also reported that it strengthened her eyesight.

A woman who needed to find courage and determination in resolving her marriage problems took homeopathic E. Taking this daily helped her focus her mind, stand up for herself, and not crumble in the face of overwhelming aggression. She was able to remain in contact with her deeper Self and stand up for what she felt to be her rights. This gave her time to reflect on how she had given her power to her husband and started the process of helping her reclaim her Self.

GREEN AND THE NOTE F

Green is the most neutral of all colors, being neither hot nor cold. It sits in the middle of the spectrum and offers respite from the heat of red, orange, and yellow and the chill of blue, purple, and violet. It is the most prevalent color in nature, and it relates to nature's healing power, bringing ease and rest to frayed nerves. Green and the note F correspond to the heart chakra, and they are associated with the transpersonal issues of love, joy, peace, and unity.

People who do well with these two remedies, together or separately, are those who are undergoing volatile change and need emotional balance in their lives. These are the most balanced and neutral of all remedies. These remedies are also good for people who are resistant to change and seek or need stability.

In the provings, both the color and the note bestowed a deep sense of peace on people who were restless and out of sorts. They soothed fractious nerves when people felt agitated, providing both relaxation and tranquility. Some provers reported restorative sleep as well. When taking the remedies, people felt at ease in tense situations, with no need to hurry. The remedies also helped to relieve pain in the lumbar region of the back and behind the heart.

Green and the note F correspond to the emotions of love and are linked with the planet Venus, which is associated with love and beauty. Green was worn at medieval weddings to signify love, fidelity, and peace. This color gives peace of mind and helps restore balance to ailing hearts.

Green and F are both natural detoxifying agents that release fluids from the body and help drain edematous tissue. They act as diuretics for congestive heart problems and have been used successfully for cardiac edema when given as homeopathic remedies.

Associated with the heart chakra, these remedies work together with homeopathic pink, combining natural tranquility and motherly love. The note and the color can be given together with homeopathic pink. These forces represent the totality of love, care, and unity in our lives. Pink represents the universal quality of love that transcends the baser emotions of the three lower chakras.

Green and the note F are essential energies in supporting life and can sustain our efforts toward inner growth and greater harmony. That is why they are recommended for those in need of balance and tranquility.

Green

Green is the easiest color for the eye to see. The lens of the eye focuses green light almost exactly onto the retina. It is a tonic for the eye, which explains why eye shades and sunglasses are often tinted green to ease harsh glare. Green has been used since ancient times as a respite for sore eyes. Medieval engravers kept a piece of green beryl to contemplate and relax their eyes after long hours at work, and in ancient Egypt, the green stone malachite was crushed and made into an unguent to protect the eyes.

There are many shades of green, each suggestive of one of the color's different aspects. Most common are lime green, which contains the fire of yellow, and blue-green, which carries the creative energy of indigo and the stillness and detachment of turquoise.

Green has a duplicity at both the physical and emotional levels. It is both the color of life and the color of decay. It is associated with nausea, poison, envy, and jealousy. It is also the color of rebirth in spring and eternal peace. Its dual nature is linked with its ability to fit at both the top part of the visible spectrum and at the bottom part. It is made from a mixture of yellow and blue and is known as a secondary color because it is made of two primary colors.

As the energy of decay, plants do not grow well under green light. Fluids drain out of them, they become lifeless, and they begin to rot and decay. Green is also associated with infection in the body, and when this color is administered in homeopathic potency, it helps drain the body of pus and poisons. When given during one woman's menstruation, she reported passing large clots along with copious urination. In the provings, green was noted for symptom of frequent urination, which several provers experienced. Green is an excellent diuretic, eliminating toxins from the body. It is used for cardiac and cellular edema.

The Note F

The note F represents the qualities of love and peace at the higher level of the astral plane, where desires can be quelled and aversions soothed. It helps bring balance to the emotions, which, if not disciplined, create damage and drama. F works on the heart chakra by helping us value what and whom we love. It helps us reflect on the nature of love in our life and gives us the ability to hold love as the central theme of our life. It stimulates the intelligence of the heart to be thoughtful and introspective. It serves higher consciousness by creating the platform for us to affirm our worth and honor our choices for love.

Green and F Uses

Here are ways to use green for physical, emotional, and mental issues.

PHYSICAL PROBLEMS

Green and F have been used successfully to drain excess fluid from the body. They act as a diuretic and help with edema, inflammation, and congestion. These remedies have been used to soothe PMS symptoms, such as when women develop engorged breasts, retain fluid in the ankles and belly, or feel highly emotional. They can be used for inflammation of the testicles or breasts and for soft tissue swelling. Both remedies can be used for both tired eyes and for headaches where there is a feeling of congestion.

Green can help women who have cystic breasts. It helps ease pain in the left breast. It has also been used, along with other heart remedies, for congestive heart failure to tonify the heart and stop fluid retention. The relief is quick, but not long-lasting.

F has been used to ease stressed nerves and provide a sense of deep tranquility after an emotional upset. It helps a person relax and calm down.

Contraindications: If there has been a serious loss of fluid from diarrhea, vomiting, or kidney failure, Green or F would not be indicated. These remedies should not be given at night since patients may need to urinate frequently.

■ EMOTIONAL ISSUES

Green and F have been used successfully on patients who have a serious lack of equilibrium in their emotional lives, who barely manage to cope with problematic situations, whose inner resources are drained, and who are tired and exhausted. It is especially good for people undergoing major life changes. Green and F help restore emotional balance and provide an opportunity to detach.

These remedies are good for fatigue and can be used whenever people are overly tired, overworked, and have trouble attaining a restful state. They help to restore peace and harmony to a stressed economy.

Contraindications: Green and F should not be given to people who need stimulation, as they are more of a tranquilizer and sedative than a stimulator. They are not to be given late at night because they may encourage urination.

■ MENTAL ISSUES

Green and F are excellent for people who suffer from nervous tension. They are good for those who are high strung and hysterical. Since they can soothe shattered nerves, these remedies help create a more balanced nervous system so that a person can think clearly and develop positive impulses. They make a person feel happier.

Contraindications: Green and F should not be given to indolent people who need energy. Again, they are not indicated for night use because of their diuretic effect.

Green and F Essence

Green and F essentially provide balance and harmony. They help restore energy to people who are exhausted and worn down without overstimulating their bodies. These remedies help a body release fluid, which is another form of retained energy. They give the heart stability and ease distress throughout the mind, body, and spirit. Since they relate so closely to the heart chakra, they are associated with the qualities of love, friendship, family, unity, and joy, and can help when life becomes stressful.

Homeopathic Remedies Related to Green and F

Homeopathic remedies that correspond most accurately to green and F are *Thuja, Craetegus*, cactus, China, Cuprum, and chrome. Aurum relates to the heart, as do *Digitalis, Hydrastis*, and *Anacardium.*

Green and F Cases

Here are cases using green and F to give you examples of how these remedies may be applied.

CASE ONE: HOMEOPATHIC GREEN

Homeopathic green helped a woman with pulmonary edema who suffered from heart pains and shortness of breath. Within a day of taking this remedy, she reported being better able to take in oxygen and felt less agitated about her condition. She had enough stamina to participate in activities that she had not been able to do for several years. She continues to take green whenever she feels her heart is taxed.

■ CASE TWO: HOMEOPATHIC F

A driven businesswoman who was constantly on the go took homeopathic F. It gave her an opportunity to relax, rest, and enjoy herself. She described it as "tranquility, gentleness, softness, misty, acceptance, and pleasant." She took the remedy whenever she felt agitated and irritable, and it helped soothe her nerves so she could experience something other than her driven behavior.

■ CASE THREE: HOMEOPATHIC GREEN

Homeopathic green was given to a young woman who suffered from asthma and shortness of breath. After a single dose of green 30C, she felt she could breathe more freely. She kept the color with her and used it instead of her inhaler. There were many times when this worked for her. She continued to take green along with a constitutional homeopathic remedy suited for asthma.

■ CASE FOUR: HOMEOPATHIC F

Homeopathic F was used to help a very serious child stop worrying about his grades in school. He experienced a deep, nagging anxiety whenever he went to school. The remedy calmed him and helped him to relax. He said he knew he'd pass in school because he studied and understood the material. After the remedy, he was calmer and began to enjoy extracurricular activities. The remedy was repeated whenever the old pattern of fretting before an exam returned.

TURQUOISE AND THE NOTE G

Turquoise is a name the French used to describe the beautiful sea around the Turkish coast. Turquoise and the note G represent creativity and self-expression. They correspond to the throat chakra and represent our innate ability to express ourselves, communicate our truth, and tap into our willpower.

This color and note are associated with spiritual values and healing. Many churches are painted terra-cotta and turquoise, and much heartfelt music is written in the note of G. Santa Sophia, the great mosque in Istanbul, is made of thousands of tiny turquoise mosaics. Often the muezzin, who calls the faithful to prayer in Islam, chants in G. Turquoise and G are linked with the vast expanse of sea and sky, which engender feelings of beauty, depth, and freedom. These are the color and sound used most often in spiritual healing to connect people with their souls.

Turquoise and the note G have a calming effect on the body and are said to be able to bring down high blood pressure. These remedies are best used when people are able to relax and have time to express themselves creatively.

This color and sound nourish the soul forces working in the throat chakra. When worn as an ornament, a turquoise stone is thought to enhance creativity and promote healing. The note G opens the channel to hearing your inner voice. Turquoise and G both show a strong connection with the mouth and throat also. One prover developed a tooth abscess while proving this color remedy, which, in homeopathic terms, suggests that it could heal this condition. Turquoise has been used for this as well as for mouth ulcers, problems with the tongue and teeth, and an ulcerated throat.

Turquoise

Turquoise and pale blue are the colors most often chosen to express beauty in clothing and decoration. The Virgin Mary's cloak was reputed to have been pale blue, and she is often depicted as the Queen of Heaven wearing her blue cloak. Turqoise and pale blue are considered the same vibration in terms of the chakras.

The supreme Greek and Roman gods, Zeus and Jupiter, are represented by turquoise. It is associated with spirituality in the Native American and Tibetan traditions. Both cultures highly prize the stone, which they frequently use in rituals. They say it represents heaven and earth in one substance. The color has been linked with royalty and led to the term "blue bloods."

In the provings, turquoise appeared to have a definite link with excess catarrh, which diminished when turquoise was taken. For example, a large, overweight woman began to lose weight while on the remedy. It is possible this color remedy stimulated her sluggish thyroid gland.

The Note G

Affiliated with the throat chakra, G helps people speak up for themselves and express their truth. Wherever they have felt unwilling or unable to speak up and ask or demand what they felt they needed, this remedy supported their inner process. G allows the energy of self-expression to be communicated in a thoughtful and mindful way. It helps people think about what they want to say. It helps people gather the will necessary to move forward in life. Musicians who have used homeopathic G have reported that their music became more attuned and creative, their voice clearer, and their expression more open and vivid.

Turquoise and G Uses

Here are ways to use turquoise and G in healing.

▨ PHYSICAL PROBLEMS

Turquoise and G can be used to heal inflammation, particularly around the throat and mouth area. These remedies can help clear up a cold or sore throat quickly. They help balance the thyroid and parathyroid, whether underactive or overactive, and can be given along with other deep-acting homeopathic remedies, including Thyroidinium. Turquoise and G are good for obesity when the thyroid is underactive and the patient has low energy, tires easily, and is apathetic.

These remedies also can be used for teeth and gum problems, and they work successfully in alleviating toothache. They can be considered for mouth ulcers, ear infections, sore throat, and bronchial inflammations.

Contraindications: Turquoise and G are not recommended for a person currently taking drugs or antibiotics. It would be best to wait for a few weeks until these drugs have left the system. They can be given both at night and during the day.

▨ EMOTIONAL ISSUES

Turquoise and G can be given to people who have problems with self-expression. They open the throat chakra so that a person feels comfortable expressing their truth, their feelings, and their intentions. These remedies create healing on the emotional level by releasing pent-up emotional tension, and allowing it to flow freely into words or creative outlets. They stimulate communication skills and strengthen people's ability to speak up for themselves. Musicians, artists, and people who are sensitive to the inner meaning of life have benefited from taking turquoise and G, both separately and together. Turquoise has been helpful for singers and people who speak publicly.

Drugs, overeating, smoking, and drink weaken the throat, and this, in turn, weakens the will. Any time the will needs to be engaged to achieve some task and is weak or shows decreased function, these remedies are indicated. For instance, if someone wants to quit smoking, begin a diet, or reject any other personal addiction, turquoise or G would strengthen their resolve.

Contraindications: These remedies are not a substitute for communication, but they do help resolve tension where it is blocked.

▒ MENTAL AND SPIRITUAL ISSUES

Turquoise and G relate to a person's ability to hear and express their truth. These remedies can help people who resist speaking up for themselves, or those who fear repercussions. They may also aid people who have very fixed ideas and have trouble hearing the opinions or feelings of others. They open our channel for hearing as well as expressing our truth. These remedies work to strengthen the will so a person can clearly express their intentions.

People who are very critical of others, who gossip and speak maliciously, can benefit from this color and note. Since so much negative energy is channeled through the throat, this color and note strengthen it and make it less likely that energy will drain away and dissipate into negativity. These remedies are good for anyone who has problems differentiating the truth.

Contraindications: None.

Turquoise and G Essence

The essence of turquoise and the note G is their ability to stimulate the expression of truth, both the higher truth of God and our personal expression of it. They stimulate our creativity and clear a path for us to express ourselves in the highest and most joyful ways. They help define a person's individuality by strengthening their will. They work on the throat chakra and are associated with all the organs of speech, hearing, and ingestion.

Homeopathic Remedies Related to Turquoise and G

Turquoise relates to the homeopathic remedies of alumina, stannum, *Ignatia*, causticum, aconite, argentum, Tuberculinum, beryllium, lithium, phosphorus, and *Caladium*.

Turquoise and G Cases

Here are cases that describe how these remedies have been used in healing.

CASE ONE: HOMEOPATHIC TURQUOISE

Homeopathic turquoise was given to a young man suffering from severe throat pain, which had been allopathically suppressed with several rounds of antibiotics. He was also very suppressed in his personal emotional expression and almost never became angered or showed irritation unless pushed to the wall. He turned his anger inward and suffered from recurring throat troubles. The remedy was repeated whenever he had a sore throat. It helped him express himself better and stopped ulceration.

CASE TWO: HOMEOPATHIC G

Homeopathic G was used to help a woman who suffered from lack of trust. It supported her to cultivate trust in herself and to decipher what was good from what was not. It helped her differentiate what might look good but was not what she needed. This remedy has that level of subtleness to it. It works on fine levels of discernment and differentiation so people become more aware of good choices for themselves. Homeopathic G has been used to clear the ears of blocked energy so they can open to the truth.

CASE THREE: HOMEOPATHIC TURQUOISE

Homeopathic turquoise was given, along with homeopathic Thyroidinium, to a woman with severe thyroid problems. It helped stabilize her and gave her more courage to speak up for herself. She had been strictly suppressed in her self-expression for many years and never felt free to speak her truth. The remedy worked both physically and emotionally.

CASE FOUR: HOMEOPATHIC G

Homeopathic G helped a woman who was very stuck in a limited vision of her life following a tragic accident. She didn't know how to move forward or how to find pleasure in creative pursuits. This remedy opened a channel for creativity to flow and gave her a stronger sense of freedom.

INDIGO AND THE NOTE A

Indigo is a color of beauty and grace. It carries the energy of the cosmos in it and is reminiscent of an evening sky on a winter day. This energy is both cool and detached. It symbolizes the intellect of the mind and detachment from the emotions. Indigo and the note A are used for healing the mind and the senses, relieving what is inflamed and impassioned. Indigo and the note A relate to the brow chakra, or, as it is known in yoga, the control center. The brow chakra is the seat of the pituitary gland, which stimulates growth and controls reproductive cycles.

This color and note have the ability to lower blood pressure, cool a fever, and enhance clarity and lucidity. The color and note both work to promote detachment from overheated emotions. Indigo and the note A are closely associated with the qualities of wisdom, discernment, knowledge, imagination, and intuition. These are the qualities of the brow chakra.

Indigo and the note A represent the energy of universal truth. This energy may be slightly cold and a little merciless, but it is able to cleanse and calm the spirit by cooling the passions that inflame the mind. If these remedies are used too much, they may destabilize people by detaching their spirits from their bodies. This energy can keep people fixed in the realm of the mind, where they remain in their intellect and forget the world around them.

Indigo and A both calm frayed nerves and anxious states. When people are too strongly engrossed or engaged in their problems, these remedies promote cool, unemotional mental clarity and control. This can help people step back from a menacing situation and reevaluate their possibilities, better able to see what is wholesome and good. This discernment is particularly strong with homeopathic A.

These remedies are not suited to anyone suffering from depression because they are too cool and detached. These people need hotter colors and lower notes, which will reanimate their ability to feel, not remedies that detach them from their feelings. The coolness of indigo and the note A help when a person wants to think clearly and express their ideas fluently.

Indigo is used to tonify the lymph, and it works well on mucous surfaces to remove inflammation. The note A soothes and helps regenerate life energy. Both remedies give a feeling of exhilaration and courage, which can increase physical strength. They act as a tonic for general health.

At a psychological level, Indigo and A can be used to cleanse and clear the body's psychic currents. They can purify and stabilize fear and repressed feelings. Indigo and A are useful for people who need to create healthy boundaries to protect them from intrusive people and experiences. These remedies give a clear mental framework and help people resolve emotional difficulties by thinking with greater clarity and in a more expanded way.

Both the color and the note stimulate the senses and can be used with eye, ear, and nose problems. They help clear headaches and soothe itchy scalps. They are both best given at night or early in the morning when the light is still a deep blue. They have a strong relationship with dawn and dusk, when the sky is a beautiful shade of indigo.

Indigo

Indigo is an anesthetic, providing soothing and cooling relief from the pain and irritation of inflammation. It is known as the universal healing color. It is ethereal, more a color of the intellect than the passions.

While on indigo, one of the provers had a sense of things being very chaotic, and she couldn't find obvious things she had left in front of her. She made writing mistakes and felt very disoriented for the first hour after taking the remedy. This suggests, in the homeopathic fashion of like curing like, that indigo could be useful for people with dyslexia and confused states of mind. The remedy also seemed to produce a clear picture of mental control, and those who took it in the provings felt they could control their lives with a greater degree of conscious mastery.

The Note A

The note A has been used for helping with long periods of concentration, when the mind can become weary and tired. It stimulates thinking and promotes focus. This remedy is excellent before taking an exam or writing a report. The note A helps us reflect on our problems so that we can find wholesome solutions to them. It helps us think in a positive and holistic way about who we are and what we are doing. If there is some issue that needs resolution, this remedy helps a person look at the bigger picture without getting emotionally tied up or becoming afraid of looking at the realm of possibilities.

Indigo and A Uses

Here are ways these remedies can be used for healing.

▩ PHYSICAL PROBLEMS

Indigo and A act as an anesthetic and help relieve pain. They are natural blood purifiers and help alleviate lymphatic congestion that causes inflammation. Both can be used effectively for swollen joints, boils or carbuncles, or skin irritation, or to soothe the internal organs. Indigo is useful for congestive problems in the pelvis, and is even considered for sterility problems in both men and women. It is used for mental instability, fever, and tuberculosis, and it has been useful in treating asthma, epilepsy, and chronic diseases with degeneration.

Contraindications: None. Remember, these remedies cool and soothe; they do not stimulate or energize.

▩ EMOTIONAL ISSUES

Indigo and A have a profound influence on calming the emotions. They are good for anxiety and fearful states or when the emotions run high. They cool, clarify, focus the mind, and relax emotional states where people become hysterical or overly involved in other people's problems. These remedies support detachment and ground a person in realistic thinking. People find they are more analytical as well as more observant on these remedies. They are also good for insane and agitated states, when people are unable to take conscious control of their actions and speech.

The note A is more mentally oriented than indigo, and it supports people in sorting through their emotional baggage. It helps people think about their lives and seek out what is important to them and what they wish to accomplish.

Contraindications: Neither of these remedies is good for depressed states and can make a person more depressed and dissociated from their feelings and body. Be aware of this before prescribing to people on antidepressants.

■ MENTAL AND SPIRITUAL ISSUES
Indigo and A are very good at helping a person organize their thoughts. They represent mentality and help the mind elucidate matters that weigh heavily. They are good tonics for tired and weary minds, and they help restore balance where clarity has been lost.

Contraindications: These remedies are not suggested for people who analyze constantly and who are always in their heads. It would only accentuate that tendency.

Indigo and A Essence
Indigo and A are essentially coolants, and they bring order to strongly heated and chaotic states, whether physical, emotional, or mental. They assist the mind in maintaining control. Their clear, soothing energy nurtures consciousness, wisdom, truth, and integrity.

Homeopathic Remedies Related to Indigo and A
Indigo and A correspond with the anterior and posterior pituitary. Sepia, lithium, cobalt, *Lachesis, Crotalus,* belladonna, Cuprum, picric acid, phosphorus, and camphor are all the homeopathic remedies that relate to indigo.

Indigo and A Cases

Here are cases that describe how these remedies are used in healing.

■ CASE ONE: HOMEOPATHIC INDIGO

A man who was in a professional bind, who was emotional and fearful, used homeopathic indigo. He was being harassed by a female colleague and didn't know how to extricate himself from the situation. The color remedy opened the channels of his mind so he could think clearly and creatively. Within a few days, his approach to the situation had changed, and he felt free. Previously, he had been only reactive. The situation resolved itself once he was detached enough to look at it clearly.

■ CASE TWO: HOMEOPATHIC A

Homeopathic A was given to a woman who was always mothering her husband. He was rude and difficult and remained immature as long as she invested her life force in "fixing" him. When it came time to think about her life and what she wanted to do for herself, this remedy gave her focus and intent. She did not prevaricate, but became very clear about what she wanted to do. When she began to focus on her own life, her husband began to mature.

■ CASE THREE: HOMEOPATHIC INDIGO

Homeopathic indigo was used to support a woman who had cataracts, hyperthyroidism with bulging eyes, and high blood pressure. This remedy soothed, cooled, and relaxed her inflamed eyes. It helped lower her blood pressure and relax her overly active mind.

■ CASE FOUR: HOMEOPATHIC A

Homeopathic A helped ease the mental tension and fear a woman had regarding making important decisions about her family. It helped her be more detached, realistic, and clear about the various opportunities for her and her children and what she could realistically expect from the changes she was putting into place. This sound remedy eliminated her fear and helped her face her challenge. It opened her ability to think clearly about her situation.

VIOLET AND THE NOTE B

Violet is a mystical color that represents spirituality and beauty. It is soft, inviting, and very gentle. This color and the musical note B are associated with serenity, beauty, and the realm of spirit. They work on the crown chakra, located at the top of the head. They link the personality, or smaller self, with the Source, also known as the Higher Self. They both enhance our intimate relationship with our higher nature, where that place of "peace beyond all peace" can be experienced. This is the place of inner stillness and quiet where the Self abides, deep within our being.

Violet and B soothe and bring comfort to the soul forces, and they also act as an anesthetic and purifier on the physical level. However, violet can create confusion and dissonance for the ego, and it requires a well-grounded person to stay anchored in himself or herself when taking this remedy.

Violet and B are associated with the pineal gland, located in the top of the skull. Scientists are still baffled by its function. Esoteric healers and Asian teachers share the belief that this gland's function is to open the spiritual center, known as the crown chakra. The pineal gland responds to light similar to the way an eye does. It is made of tiny light-sensitive rods and cones. This light sensitivity is thought to control many physical functions, such as women's menstruation and reproductive cycles. Other pineal functions include the feeling of jet lag, fatigue associated with our intake of light, and the production of melatonin.

Tibetan lamas practice specific yoga postures and say mudras and prayers that stimulate the pineal gland to secrete an essence they call nectar, a substance reputed to enhance feelings of ecstasy and bliss. This takes many years of devotion and practice.

Violet and B created an "otherworldly feeling" for many of the provers. Violet created nausea, disorientation, and headache in some provers, which means it would be useful in treating those conditions in people who suffered from these symptoms. It has been used to palliate pain in cancer care, giving relief and peace.

Violet and B can be used by the elderly, as it is a vibration to which they are more closely attuned. They are also good for people who have difficulty finding a spiritual path in life. These remedies help them attune to a greater understanding of their purpose in life, as well as develop a more refined sense of beauty and serenity.

Both remedies can be used to treat epileptic seizures and alcoholism, along with deeper-acting homeopathic remedies. Violet was given to an artist who was unable to see or paint violet or purple until he took the remedy. He suffered from seizures and was a recovering alcoholic. Whenever he attempted to paint these colors, they appeared as a muddy brown. After taking homeopathic violet, he was able to paint a natural violet color.

It has been found that people may lose their sense of ego identity when exposed to too much violet or B. If people are not grounded in their personal identity, they easily become susceptible to the influence of others. They find it difficult to make decisions and be affirmative, and they can become touchy and irritable. They can become ungrounded in their spirituality and afraid of moving forward. However, violet is a gentle color and can give great comfort to those who are overly sensitive.

Violet

It is traditionally felt that violet represents the spiritual aspect and purple stands for the temporal element of power represented by the Catholic Church. Purple was a color reserved only for nobility, both in ancient Rome and Byzantium. It was very expensive to make and required the use of thousands of tiny mollusks to obtain the color. The expression "to the purple born" comes from Byzantium, where all queens were required to give birth to future emperors in a room completely swathed in purple silk. This may have actually been quite hygienic, as purple and violet are both anesthetics. Purple is now worn by high-ranking officials in the Catholic Church at specific times during the liturgical year.

Violet is found in nature in beautiful spring and summer flowers. It is seldom seen in the animal kingdom, except as a marker of the Brown Recluse spider, but in the mineral world it can be found in manganese, magnesium, amethyst, and fluorine. Violet can enhance awareness when used in crystal healing and helps to open the spiritual centers.

A highly evolved spiritual teacher in India who complained of chronic pain in his feet and legs was treated with homeopathic violet. He was given violet 6X in a split dose, and all of his pain disappeared. He resonated with the violet ray so strongly it seemed to be the best medicine to give him.

Violet has also been used by headache sufferers who were troubled by spiritual and ethical problems. These sufferers had conflicts between higher spiritual ideals and their emotions. Violet relieved the pain, and the headaches never reoccurred.

The Note B

The note B is very gentle and tender. The people who proved the note B came away with a very gentle, loving feeling. They were not very determined or aggressive and acted quiet, ungrounded, and submissive in their approach to situations and other people. They were easily irritated when they could not make up their minds. This indicates that B could aid people who dither and are passive in their approach to life.

The provers of violet did not want to connect with their problems, understand difficult challenges, or get involved. They wanted to be left alone to watch fantasy videos and stay secluded. Conversely, this remedy can assist with shyness and timidity and when people are frightened of exposing themselves to strangers and act introverted. It helps people feel spiritually connected and part of a greater whole and supports people on their spiritual path.

Violet and B Uses

Here is how violet and B can be used for healing.

PHYSICAL PROBLEMS

Violet and B, because of their connection with the crown chakra, can be used to help brain disorders, such as alcoholism, epilepsy, and neurosis. They are particularly good for stopping pain and can be used for menstrual cramps, headaches, and any pain around the head and shoulder area.

Contraindications: Violet could make people who are too sensitive feel uneasy and irritable. Magenta may have better results, as it carries the red and green rays. It is suggested that if there is mental or emotional instability, a small amount of violet can be used, but once the patient becomes restless or uneasy, it is best to stop the treatment. Violet and B are best given at night.

EMOTIONAL ISSUES

Violet can be used to open realms of spiritual understanding, ease impacted emotions, and bring the gift of inner peace. It soothes nervous conditions in which a person feels fractious and out of sorts. Violet and B can bring emotional stability to violent minds and relief to neurotic states of anxiety and chronic worry.

Contraindications: These remedies should be used in limited dosage. The remedies can be used alone or together, with time for observing the patient's response before giving a second dose. Caution should be used with hypersensitive people or people who are taking prescription medication.

MENTAL AND SPIRITUAL ISSUES

Violet and B give a person a spiritual outlook on life. They can both ease egotistical streaks and narcissistic tendencies. These remedies can be useful for anyone trying to grow emotionally. However, too strong an identification with the spiritual plane can limit a person's individuation, or healthy ego development. Violet and B can cause a person to surrender their ego too readily. Finding a balance and staying grounded with this color is important.

Contraindications: Use judiciously with people who have a weak ego or who are taking prescription medication. They can become very sensitized, even temporarily insane, from too much violet light.

Violet and B Essence

Violet and B are energy fields that connect us to our higher spiritual nature. They both reflect the divine light within us and help us connect to the beauty around us and our innate serenity. They are gentle and healing, cleansing a person's aura and attuning them to the spiritual aspects of life.

Homeopathic Remedies Related to Violet and B

The magnesium remedies relate to Violet and B, as does manganeum. These remedies focus on crown chakra issues and have a strong effect on inner stability, the alleviation of pain, and well-being. Hydrogen corresponds to the violet ray, as do DNA and other life-building substances. Homeopathic iris vericolor and pansy also correspond to this field. Violet fluorine and amethyst gem remedies also carry this vibration.

Violet and B Cases

Here are cases that describe how violet and B have been used in healing.

CASE ONE: HOMEOPATHIC VIOLET

Homeopathic violet was given to a woman with chronic migraine headaches. She had suffered for over forty years, and the intensity of her pain was increasing, as was the frequency of her attacks. She was taken off her strong medication, which failed to relieve her symptoms. After a week of detoxification with homeopathic remedies, she took violet 30C. This helped relieve her intense pain. Deep-acting homeopathic remedies slowed the frequency of her attacks. She continues to take this color remedy when she feels stressed or feels the possibility of a headache.

CASE TWO: HOMEOPATHIC B

Homeopathic B was given to a very passive and spiritual woman who appeared afraid of life. It helped her incarnate her spirit more fully and embody herself on the material plane. It helped her find her voice, as well as her courage. She continued to take the remedy whenever she felt herself disconnect from life.

CASE THREE: HOMEOPATHIC VIOLET

Homeopathic violet was given to a woman who had daily backache from an injury and suffered chronic pain and insomnia. The pain kept her awake at night. This remedy relaxed her and allowed her to sleep. It gave her tranquility and relieved her pain.

CASE FOUR: HOMEOPATHIC B

Homeopathic B helped a very aggressive man calm down and think about the effect his anger had on the people around him. He was both menacing and threatening, but didn't see this in himself. This remedy soothed his nerves and made him much more agreeable to be with.

PINK (NO MUSICAL NOTE APPLIES)

Pink is the color of joy and universal mother love. It is a favorite color with young children and is associated with the heart chakra. Pink is closely associated with gentleness, sweetness, and naïveté. It represents the purity and innocence of the human heart and helps open our capacity to give and receive love. Pink is found in the aura of babies, visible through Kirlian photography. It is the color that reflects the joy of life.

Pink is about inner and outer rosiness, and it indicates that there is vitality and life within us. Pink has been associated with little girls, but is now a color that is finding its place in men's fashions. When it is worn or used in decoration, it is linked with the softer, sweeter side of life. This color is positive, loving, and a sign of the purity and innocence of the human heart. It represents joy and tenderness.

In the provings of pink, all the provers had a dream associated with motherhood. They dreamed that either they were physically close to their mothers or were pregnant, giving birth, or holding a baby. This was not specific to women; men also had dreams of being held by their mothers or loved and cherished by their mothers. These dreams about mother love suggest that pink be used when we feel disconnected from love.

In the provings, pink also made everyone feel well. People found their problems were less acute, and they could manage them better. They all reported feeling well in themselves. Even provers who had serious family, financial, or health problems responded well while on the remedy. It also had a specific physical action on skin problems, relieving dry eczema, acne, and skin rash. These conditions, at an esoteric level, are thought to be reflections of feeling unloved.

Pink Uses

This is how pink can be used in healing.

▨ PHYSICAL PROBLEMS

Pink can be used for heart problems and is excellent for reviving vitality without the aggressive energy of red or orange. It can help people overcome shock, such as the trauma of childbirth, injury, or grief. It is a general toner and helps people through difficult times of change when they feel tired, fed up, or exhausted. Pink can be used for any skin condition, which suggests a person may be somatizing feelings of rejection and being unloved into physical pathology.

Contraindications: None.

▨ EMOTIONAL ISSUES

Pink is associated with love. Whenever there is a hardening or an emotional closing down, this color remedy can be used to add a soft and gentle quality to a person's life. It is good for heartache, loss, and emotional suffering, especially in association with the loss of feminine love. Pink is not just a woman's remedy. It can be given to either sex at any age, wherever there is grief or loss of love. When combined with orange, it adds vitality and a sense of joy to any situation.

Contraindications: None.

Pink can add a soft emotional element to the harsh light of the mind. It offers a sweetness and a refreshing quality to mental activity.

Contraindications: None.

Pink Essence

Pink is the color of love. It offers us the bloom of roses, the sweetness of youth, and the joy of the heart. It suggests something childlike in us that relates to eternal youth, innocence, and motherhood. It fills us with a sweet, gentle, and humorous light.

Homeopathic Remedies Related to Pink

Related homeopathic remedies include ignatia, the muriaticums, Kali Phos., Phos. Ac., pulsatilla, and *Impatiens.* The milk remedies would also correspond to pink, as they promote self-love.

Pink Cases

Here are cases that show how pink can be used in healing.

■ CASE ONE: HOMEOPATHIC PINK

An elderly woman who had lost her son recently and whose husband was suffering from Alzheimer's was heavy with grief and depleted physically, with a weak heart. She took pink every night, and it gave her profound relief from her sorrows. She created a pink room—replete with a pink rocking chair—knitted a pink shawl, and kept her remedy in a pink box. It became part of her nightly ritual to take her remedy in her pink environment.

■ CASE TWO: HOMEOPATHIC PINK

An angry woman who had recently divorced and was unhappy with her life found relief from her emotions by taking pink 30C once a week. It reminded her of what she really wanted in her life, which was love, ease, and joy.

■ CASE THREE: HOMEOPATHIC PINK

A seventeen-year-old autistic girl was given pink 12C twice a week and began to ask for things she wanted. She was later given pink 12C in combination with orange 30C and started to become more playful, less introverted, and better able to connect with the world around her.

■ CASE FOUR: HOMEOPATHIC PINK

A young woman was given pink 30C by her mother after a romantic relationship broke up. This calmed her and gave her peace of mind. She was able to reflect on the relationship and deal with her grief without dramatic acting out and without shrinking away from the world, thinking it had been her fault. Her mother was mindful of her daughter's grief, but also very struck with how she handled herself. She never had to repeat the remedy.

MAGENTA AND THE NOTE HIGH C

Magenta is a regal color. Dr. Rudolf Steiner calls it the color of ultimate creativity. The color is a mixture of green, red, and violet, and it encompasses the energy of red's life force; green's peace, harmony, and neutrality; and violet's serenity and beauty.

Magenta and high C correspond to the alta major chakra, which sits about a foot above the crown chakra. This energy center is concerned with our higher purpose in life. This chakra represents the collective unconscious and the bonds of humanity that make us all one.

Magenta

Magenta is reserved for special occasions and creative ventures. Whenever we want a depth of understanding that supports our deepest spiritual nature, homeopathic magenta is the color of choice.

The esoteric issues of the alta major chakra correspond to the contracts made with our guardian spirits before incarnation. This color links us to the distant memory of past lives and also to the spiritual realm, where guidance, protection, and love are given to us.

In the provings, homeopathic magenta helped people gain insight into their problems. It added a spiritual dimension to the way they perceived situations. It seemed to elevate those who were too grounded in their thinking, and ground those who were too "airy" in their approach to life.

Magenta has been given to victims of abuse and to children who had neglectful parents. In all cases, it helped the person reestablish links with their Higher Self and gain wisdom and insight.

Magenta is used in color healing to stimulate a person's adrenals, heart, and sexuality because it is made in part with red. Magenta is said to strengthen the heart muscles and stabilize the heart rhythm. This color should be considered whenever there is fluid retention and also when the patient may need the extra vitality that they would receive from red. It can be considered a tonic for elderly people. Also, it is felt that many female disorders are helped by magenta. It has a diuretic effect as well, because of the green component, and helps release excess fluid from the system.

This color remedy was given to a woman who had developed weeping sores on both her legs at a crisis point in her thirty-year marriage. She had not responded to any other remedies. She could not see a future for herself if she stayed in her marriage, and she did not know what to do. This color helped her focus and helped her find a horizon. When she took the remedy, her wounds began to heal and she found the sense of freedom she needed to think about what she wanted from life.

The Note High C

The note high C corresponds to the alta major chakra. It is the end of one scale and the beginning of another. It provides a way of thinking about spiritual realities, and it encompasses past, present, and future in its totality. It offers a visionary way of thinking, with both sides of the brain involved, and helps a person maintain a clear horizon with hope, trust, and faith in the future. High C is more than just the energy of this center: it is the logos for it. With this note, the realms of spirit and humanity blend together. This note opens up new ways of looking at ourselves in relation to all of life, both visible and invisible.

Magenta and High C Uses

Here are ways magenta and high C are used in healing.

PHYSICAL PROBLEMS

Magenta and high C can be used as good heart tonics. They can also be used for impotency, frigidity, and low libido. These remedies help stabilize the nerves when they are stretched from too much tension. Magenta stimulates sexuality by increasing circulation and the rate at which the heart pumps blood. It can also be used as a remedy for slow or late onset of the menses, infertility, or endometriosis.

Contraindications: Magenta should not be used on hysterical patients.

EMOTIONAL ISSUES

Magenta and high C are given when a person lacks insight, or when their emotions are too strongly engaged and they need an overview of the presenting problem. These remedies suit people who have trouble envisioning a clear horizon.

Contraindications: None.

MENTAL AND SPIRITUAL ISSUES

Great thinkers gravitate to magenta and high C. These remedies awaken latent creativity and also stimulate the vital physical and sexual realms. This energy can be transmuted into creative expression. These remedies elevate thinking toward higher realms of awareness while maintaining a grounded and realistic approach to life.

Contraindications: None.

Magenta and High C Essence

The essence of magenta and high C is creativity and insight. These remedies combine the best of the vital force contained in red, the peace and tranquility of green, and the beauty and bliss of violet. They enhance our acceptance of what is universal in mankind and stimulate our creative powers.

Homeopathic Remedies Related to Magenta and High C

Strontium, the Kalis, manganese, *Digitalis*, niobium, and molybdenum are all related to magenta and high C.

Magenta and High C Cases

Here are examples of how magenta and high C can be used in healing.

▦ CASE ONE: HOMEOPATHIC MAGENTA

A young girl whose mother had been abusive and neglectful had difficulty not internalizing this bad behavior. She was given several doses of magenta 30C over a period of months and, with the help of therapy and a loving stepmother, was able to see how her mother behaved was not her fault. She went on to develop healthy friendships, attend college, and eventually marry and become a mother herself. Magenta was instrumental in freeing her from imploding her anger, helping her recognize where the blame lay for bad behavior, and, eventually, helping her to move past the events and forgive her mother.

▦ CASE TWO: HOMEOPATHIC HIGH C

A widow in her mid sixties who had forgotten how to have fun, let down her guard, and find the lighter side of life was given high C. She began to spend time doing unimportant but relaxing things and was better able to find joy and simplicity in her life.

CASE THREE: HOMEOPATHIC MAGENTA

A man contemplating divorce was given magenta 30C to take daily until he made up his mind about what he was going to do. He decided to stay in his marriage, committed to making it work, and confronted his wife about what was bothering him. They went into therapy and resolved their issues. He said the magenta helped him see clearly and not simply react to being unhappy.

CASE FOUR: HOMEOPATHIC HIGH C

An abused child who was always sad and scared felt uncomfortable around groups of people and would act obsessively or sit in silence, gazing into the distance. He was given high C and became more responsive to life: he began to lose his fear of people, come out of his tightly closed shell, and communicate his needs more clearly. He began to feel the warmth of the people who cared for him and responded affectionately.

SPECTRUM AND THE CHORD

Spectrum and the chord are compiled by using all the color remedies to create a rainbow, or spectrum, and all the musical notes to create the chord. They have a very strong affinity with immunosuppressive diseases or diseases that weaken a person's entire energetic system.

If a person's immune system is affected, these remedies can boost energy. Spectrum was first used with a fifty-six-year-old woman who suffered from full-blown AIDS. She had previously had cancer and was so depleted that she could do nothing herself. She took spectrum 12C five times daily for several weeks. After the first week, she reported that she was able to do her housework, wash her hair, and dress herself for the first time in nearly a year. She had the energy to resolve many of the issues in her life that she had ignored. She said goodbye to those she loved and had the energy, right up to the last days, to take care of herself. She lived an extra six months and had a peaceful passing. Since then, the remedy has been given to anyone with serious energy depletion problems, HIV, AIDS, or other immunosuppressive diseases, with successful results.

Spectrum

Spectrum can be given over a long period of time without aggravation, and it seems to have a restorative effect when used for times of stress and exhaustion. It can be used as a travel remedy as well and gives energy whenever it is used.

Spectrum also helps eliminate the effects of drugs (such as repeated doses of allopathic medicine) from a person's aura, and, after taking it, people have had increased levels of vitality and awareness. Any substance abuse case, where the body is weakened or depleted of vitality, will reveal an auric field that is ash or gray. Spectrum revitalizes the entire energetic system and brings color back into a person's aura. It is useful for drug rehabilitation or alcohol recovery.

The Chord

The chord inspires holistic thinking and clarity in all endeavors. Like spectrum, it is a broadly used remedy, focusing intelligence on resolution and refinement. It is given in a low potency and needs to be repeated as needed. This sound remedy can open the realms of creative thinking and help expand the way a person looks at any situation.

Spectrum and the Chord Uses

Here are ways spectrum and the chord can be used for healing.

▪ PHYSICAL PROBLEMS

Spectrum and the chord boost energy. They work in autoimmune deficiency and immunosuppressive conditions and have been used successfully with AIDS, HIV, chronic fatigue syndrome, postviral syndrome, glandular fever, alcoholism, and drug abuse. They also help with pregnancy, labor, and postpartum care. Any degenerative disease responds to these remedies because they give people energy to heal. People who have been ill a long time have more vitality with their use. This healing energy also benefits anyone with a long-term chronic disease, where severe pathology exists.

Contraindications: Spectrum should not be given at night, so as not to disturb sleep.

▪ EMOTIONAL ISSUES

Spectrum and the chord provide relief to people with nervous exhaustion and emotional upset. They help people handle change and trauma in their lives.

Contraindications: None.

▪ MENTAL AND SPIRITUAL ISSUES

Spectrum and the chord revive tired minds and are excellent to take after working with large groups of people or in other situations where energy can be drained. They establish peace and balance after long hours of engagement in a project.

Contraindications: None.

Spectrum and the Chord Essence

The essence of spectrum and the chord is the energy of all the colors and all the notes, which revitalizes a worn-out, fatigued system. These remedies contain all the vibrations within the visible spectrum and musical scale, to provide energy for a person's spirit as well as their body.

Homeopathic Remedies Related to Spectrum and the Chord

There are no relationships between spectrum and the chord and specific homeopathic remedies.

Spectrum and the Chord Cases

Here are examples of how spectrum and the chord can be used in healing.

CASE ONE: HOMEOPATHIC SPECTRUM

Spectrum was given to a man suffering from chronic fatigue syndrome. He had to quit his job and go on unemployment insurance, and he slept twelve to fourteen hours a day. His energy revived quickly and he found he had the clarity and the energy he needed to work part-time and, eventually, go back to full-time employment. He took the remedy daily for over a year.

CASE TWO: HOMEOPATHIC CHORD

The chord was given to a woman who felt confused and mentally dull from overwork. It helped her find clarity and enthusiasm for her life and supported her in making some wholesome choices for herself.

CASE THREE: HOMEOPATHIC SPECTRUM

An airline stewardess who suffered from chronic leg pain found relief taking spectrum 6X each time she flew. It helped decongest her circulation and gave her energy to do her work efficiently.

CASE FOUR: HOMEOPATHIC SPECTRUM AND CHORD

The chord was given to a young woman who had been in a serious car accident and suffered from vertigo, nausea, confusion, and asthma since her accident. The chord opened her field so she could process more energy. She began working with color and sound in a more consistent way until she felt she was fully recovered. She takes the chord when she needs mental clarity and spectrum for energy.

Afterword

Thank you for reading this book. I sincerely hope that you will derive knowledge and benefit from delving into the fascinating world of color and sound. Especially at a greatly diluted level, color and sound have tremendous healing power to work for our highest good and greater development. Color and sound are life, and they anchor us in the eternal constancy of universal and spiritual truths. It is appropriate to say that, while we are in that interim stage of being on earth, we live a colorful and resonant existence.

If you are interested in purchasing a set of homeopathic color or sound remedies, please send the following to the address below:

1. Your name and address.
2. The color or sound remedy kit you want, specifying potency. (Homeopathic color remedy sets come in 6X, 12C, and 30C. Homeopathic sound remedies come in one potency only. Because the color remedy potencies and the sound remedy potencies could differ, one from the other.)

3. A check or money order for $115 for one kit, $205 for two kits, or $310 for three kits. If you live outside the United States, please be prepared to pay additional postage and insurance.

Mail to:

Ambika Wauters
2818 N. Campbell Road, #137
Tucson, AZ 85719

All kits are sent FedEx ground in the United States or air for foreign post.

If you would like information about professional training in homeopathy at the School of Spiritual Homeopathy or wish to attend a course on homeopathic color and sound remedies, please visit www.lifeenergymedicine.com or call Ambika Wauters at 1-877-774-1812. Training sessions are offered regularly, and trained teachers can visit your community to offer workshops.

Homeopathic Potency Choices

Helios Pharmacy in Tunbridge Wells, Kent, UK, potentized the color remedies in the following potencies: 6X, 12C, and 30C; all of the kits sold by the author are in these potencies. However, Roger Savage, a UK homeopath, has taken them up to 200C, 1M, and 10M on his Ray-Potentizer machine. He has had success with the higher potencies and has found them particularly useful for acute problems.

We find that the remedies work best when kept at 30C and lower, and do not encourage people to raise the potency, because the effects need to remain short and intense. Potencies in 30C and lower give a level of protection, do not create aggravation, and are safe, gentle, and easy to manage.

All the provings were carried out using 30C potencies. The results varied as to each remedy's duration. Some symptoms disappeared and never returned, such as gallbladder colic, rheumatoid arthritis pains, and chronic rhinitis. This is interesting and suggests that the provers received doses that matched their own constitutional nature. In other words, it was the right vibration and frequency for their symptoms. The low potency of 6X, when repeated up to five times a day, has been useful for all immuno-deficiency cases.

People with significant mental and emotional symptoms who were treated with a single dose of 30C seldom needed more than the initial dose, and then only needed occasional repetitions for a few years. When it was necessary to repeat a color or sound remedy, the color or note directly higher than the first one given was often used, rather than a higher potency of the same remedy. For instance, someone whose symptoms disappeared with yellow would need green (lime green or a darker green) for symptoms that arose subsequently. A person who did well on D would then take E.

It is possible to perform muscle testing or dowse for remedies to find the right potency and then check often before repeating it. However, physical and emotional symptoms can be a better diagnostic tool than muscle testing, because they refer directly to the chakra that is out of balance.

Each potency of a color carries its own particular frequency of healing. The rule of thumb is that physical symptoms respond well to low potencies, such as 6X, and as potencies progress past 12C, the remedies heal emotional and mental states. However, there is a hierarchy of incremental change that the colors and sounds represent. For example, there is a distinct difference between a red 30C and turquoise 3X.

Careful study of the chakra system will lead to a better understanding of the problems and issues that relate to each energy center and the appropriate sound and color potencies to treat affected centers. Refining our understanding of color and sound and how they work in the human economy will also aid our grasp of the essential qualities of each potency.

The sound remedies were purposely kept at low potencies because they proved to be so powerful in the 5–7X potency range. These potencies provided sufficient stimulation to a person's energy system. When we fully understand the astral forces and how they strengthen or weaken according to our thinking, we will raise the potencies. Until then, we feel it is safer to create stability and constancy with the lower potencies. Meanwhile, we know these sound remedies encourage growth, intelligence, and consciousness as they are now.

Physical Therapeutics

COLOR & SOUND	PHYSICAL SYMPTOMS
Red and Middle C	Good for pains and irritations with joints and ligaments of the feet, ankles, knees, and hips; rectal and bowel difficulties; childbirth and postpartum care; varicose veins; piles; circulatory problems; and autoimmune deficiency diseases.
Orange and D	Good for sexual problems for both sexes, menstrual problems, lower backaches, allergies of all kinds, constipation and sluggish bowels, anorexia and eating disorders, low vitality and postoperative recovery, and autoimmune deficiency diseases.
Yellow and E	A general detoxifier; good for liver, gallbladder, stomach, and pancreas problems; absorption problems, such as ciliacs; osteoporosis; right eye vision loss; and decongestion for colds and pulmonary problems.
Green and F	A general diuretic; good for edematous tissues, especially suited for pulmonary and cardiac edema; a cardiac regulator and tonic, detoxifier, calmative, and tranquilizer.

COLOR & SOUND	PHYSICAL SYMPTOMS
Turquoise and G	A catarrhal remedy, good for sore throats and tired speaking voices; a stimulant to the thyroid and parathyroid; good for substance abuse cases where a patient wants to stop smoking, drinking, or overeating; good for neck and shoulder pain.
Indigo and A	Good for tuning the eyes, ears, and nose; a calmative, good for insomnia; an anti-inflammatory, good for sinus problems, fevers, and congestion to the head, such as migraine, head strain, or eye strain.
Violet and B	An antiseptic, good for helping wounds heal quickly; a nervous tonic, good for soothing frayed nerves; improves left eye vision; an antinausea remedy; a complement in jaundice and liver conditions.
Pink (no note applies)	Good for heart patients to ease fears and the tension of heart disease; good for new mothers to help increase milk production and attune them to motherhood; good for relieving stress.
Magenta and High C	Good for sexual, heart, and mind ailments; a tonic, good for low energy.
Spectrum and the Chord	A general tonic, good for burnout, post-viral, or trauma conditions; good for substance abuse, overwork, or emotional difficulties that drain vitality.

Emotional and Mental Therapeutics

COLOR & SOUND	EMOTIONAL & MENTAL SYMPTOMS
Red and Middle C	Good for disharmony in vital energy due to feelings of separation or feeling disconnected from a place, family, or community when links are weakened; good for suicidal and chronic depression, acute and prolonged grief, or a sense of uprooting.
Orange and D	Good for sensual and sexual difficulties, poverty consciousness, depression, mobility difficulties, and very low energy due to depressed states.
Yellow and E	Good for low ego and confidence; fearful, agitated, or angry states; and decreased intelligence, independence, and inner strength.
Green and F	Good for distress, feelings of inner conflict, avoidance of change, and a weakened spirit.

COLOR & SOUND	EMOTIONAL & MENTAL SYMPTOMS
Turquoise and G	Good for lack of creative expression, lack of willpower to complete tasks, integrity issues, malicious gossipers, liars, and timid and shy communicators.
Indigo and A	Good for unclear thinking, closed mindedness, nearsightedness, and limited thinking.
Violet and B	Good for disharmony, ungroundedness, weakened ego development, lack of a spiritual sense, egotism, chronic pain dulling perception of life, and prejudice.
Pink (no note applies)	For engaging the heart where feelings of love are weakened due to grief, disappointment, loss, and separation.
Magenta and High C	Good for low-level thinking, lack of personal creativity and originality, lack of insight, inability to change, and lack of spice of life.
Spectrum and the Chord	Good for burnout on all levels, exhaustion, tension, chronic illness, and mental funk.

Energy Assessment for the Chakras

Have the person to be assessed answer the following questions to the best of their ability. Listen to the answers carefully to determine the strength or weakness of each of their chakras. Always treat the lowest chakra first in order to create stability, grounding, and a good foundation. After one chakra heals, move on to any other centers that require attention.

▪ ROOT CHAKRA

To what extent do you:

- Know what your roots are? Do you know where your ancestors came from and what they were like as people?
- Know what you inherited from your ancestors at the physical, emotional, and mental levels?
- Have healthy models for living creatively and wholesomely?
- Believe in the right to living your own life?
- Live the life you want to live?
- Experience challenges patiently?
- Organize your life?
- Remain stable during change?
- Feel secure with life?
- Take care of yourself when under stress?

- Give your energy to others in return for security or approval?
- Act like a victim when life does not go your way?

On a scale of one to ten, ten being the highest rating and one being the lowest, how would you evaluate the following qualities in your life?

- Being patient
- Having a structure that supports you being the best you can be
- Maintaining stability
- Having security
- Being able to manifest your dreams in reality
- Being able to establish order in your life
- Being able to care for yourself

Which of these qualities would you like to cultivate to enhance your root chakra?

- Trust
- Hope
- Cleverness
- Tenacity
- Perseverance

▪ SACRAL CHAKRA

To what extent do you:

- Deserve good things in life?
- Receive the abundance that is rightfully yours?
- Find pleasure in life?
- Take time to look after your physical well-being?
- Take care of your health?
- Enjoy free time and holidays?

- Get enough rest?
- Do creative things that you enjoy?
- Regard your sexuality as important?
- Act like a martyr and forgo your happiness and pleasure?

On a scale of one to ten, ten being the highest rating and one being the lowest, how would you evaluate the following aspects of your life?

- Having a sense of well-being
- Being deserving
- Feeling pleasure
- Having abundance

Which of these qualities would you like to cultivate to develop your sacral chakra?

- Physical movement: dance, tai chi, chi gong, walking, jogging, Pilates, working out, swimming
- Ease
- Fun
- Prosperity
- Sexuality
- Sensuality

SOLAR PLEXUS CHAKRA

To what extent do you:

- Link your self-worth to what you have and what you do?
- Believe you are worthy of what you say you want?
- Believe that you are worthy simply because you exist?
- Know who you really are?
- Honor yourself?
- Feel confident about your ability to be yourself, make wholesome choices, and live independently?

- Value your freedom to make good choices?
- Fight for what you believe is yours?
- Stand up to authority?
- Know you are worthy of love, kindness, and respect?
- Act like a servant to please others?

On a scale of one to ten, ten being the highest rating and one being the lowest, how would you evaluate the following qualities and attributes in your life?

- Having a sense of direction, knowing where you are going and what you want from life
- Believing that you can have what you want
- Sensing that you are worthy and deserving of good things
- Feeling entitled to acknowledgment
- Feeling that you are a free agent to determine your own path
- Feeling confident that you can achieve what you believe in
- Feeling proud of things you have achieved in your past

Which of the following qualities would you like to cultivate to develop your solar plexus chakra?

- Self-worth
- Self-esteem
- Confidence
- Personal power
- Ability to manipulate
- Personal freedom

HEART CHAKRA

To what extent do you:

- Love who you are?
- Search for peace in your life?
- Love others unconditionally?

- Love yourself unconditionally?
- Allow love to be the guiding factor in your life?
- Receive love from the world around you?
- Give love to others?
- Feel a sense of unity with others, your community, and the planet?
- Experience a sense of brotherhood with people around you?

On a scale of one to ten, ten being the highest rating and one being the lowest, how would you evaluate the following aspects of your life?

- Feeling at peace with yourself and those around you
- Harboring resentment for the way others have treated you in the past
- Feeling that you will never find the love you seek
- Feeling you have the love you seek
- Feeling safe and secure in your personal relationships
- Feeling love for those who are and have been a part of your life
- Feeling connected to the world around you

Which of the following qualities would you like to cultivate to enhance your heart chakra?

- Unconditional love
- Unity with all life
- Inner peace

▪ THROAT CHAKRA

On a scale of one to ten, ten being the highest rating and one being the lowest, to what extent do you:

- Express your truth?
- Tune into your higher truth about a situation or other people?

- Listen to your inner guidance?
- Express your creative nature?
- Value integrity?
- Speak honestly and openly about what is important to you?
- Discipline yourself and use your will?
- Abuse yourself with tobacco, recreational drugs, allopathic medicine, or over- or undereating?
- Gossip and malign others?
- Fail to speak up when you are unhappy or hurt?

Which of the following attributes would you like to cultivate to enhance your throat chakra?

- Being gentle
- Being tender
- Being passionate
- Having a sense of unity
- Feeling a sense of brotherhood
- Being peaceful
- Being joyful
- Loving unconditionally

BROW CHAKRA

On a scale of one to ten, ten being the highest rating and one being the lowest, to what extent do you:

- Seek wisdom from the pain, separation, trauma, or loss in your life?
- Trust your intuition to give you good guidance?
- Want to learn about new things that can help you grow?
- Use your imagination to see what you want to create in your future?
- Discern who and what is for your highest good?
- See the realm of possibilities before you?

On a scale of one to ten, ten being the highest rating and one being the lowest, how developed are the following qualities in your life?

- An ability to discern who and what are for your highest good
- A sense that your intuition is one of your greatest assets
- A powerful imagination and sense of desire to see your future unfold as you imagine it to be
- A desire to find wisdom in the painful situations of your life
- A desire to seek knowledge, rather than information, for your inner development

Which of the following qualities would you like to develop to enhance your brow chakra?

- Intuition
- Wisdom
- Discernment
- Imagination
- Knowledge

CROWN CHAKRA

To what extent do you:

- See beauty in all things?
- Find what is tranquil and serene around you?
- Make a daily and regular connection with Source?
- Find the spiritual truth in the situations in which you find yourself?
- Reinforce your connection with Spirit?
- Know the oneness of all life?
- Bring healing into your life?

On a scale of one to ten, ten being the highest rating and one being the lowest, what qualities are essential for your spiritual development?

- Having inner peace
- Attaining a sense of unity
- Knowing bliss
- Being serene
- Accepting life
- Trusting your spirit
- Having faith

Which of the following matter the most to you?

- Spiritual attainment
- Oneness with your fellow humans
- Connection with the spirit realm
- Psychic ability to know the future

ALTA MAJOR CHAKRA

This field is incredibly difficult to work with, and diagnosis requires complicated questions that are beyond the scope of this exercise.

Index

Note: The letter *t* indicates a table.

Law of Cure, 41, 58
Light, using, 24

Magenta
    color qualities, 46t, 147–149, 161t
    pallative qualities, 151, 152
Miasms
    described, 71–72
    remedies associated with, 35–36
    triggers for, 47
Minerals
    earth energy and, 37
    our being and, 35
    use of, 27
Moodiness, transforming, 20
Morgan, John, 17–18

Newton, Isaac, 22, 23
Note A
    note qualities, 131–133, 161t, 163t
    pallative uses, 136, 137
Note B
    note qualities, 137–138, 140
    pallative uses, 143
Note D
    note qualities, 105, 160t, 163t
    pallative uses, 109–110
Note E
    note qualities, 110–111, 160t, 162t
    pallative uses, 117, 118
Note F
    note qualities, 118–121, 160t, 162t
    pallative uses, 123, 124
Note G
    note qualities, 126–127, 129,
        160t, 163t
    pallative uses, 130
Note high C
    note qualities, 149–150, 161t, 163t
    pallative uses, 151, 152

Note middle C, 93–95
    note qualities, 93–95, 160t, 162t
    palliative uses, 95–100

O'Malley, Monica, 19–20
Orange
    color qualities, 46t, 103–105,
        160t, 162t
    pallative qualities, 105–108

Pancreas, 58
Physical body, 35–37. See also
        specific colors
Physical therapeutics, 160–161t
Pink
    color qualities, 46t, 144–146,
        160t, 163t
    pallative uses, 146–147
Pituitary gland, 10
Poisons, use of, 4–5
Proving process, 9–11, 12–14

Red
    color qualities, 46t, 88–93,
        160t, 162t
    pallative uses, 95–100
Root chakra, 45t. See also Root/
        sacral chakra
    energy assessment for, 166–167
Root/sacral chakra, 12, 44, 47, 48,
        59–62, 69–73

Sacral chakra, 45t. See also Root/
        sacral chakra
    energy assessment for, 167–168
School of Spiritual Homeopathy,
        7, 11
Self-awareness, 21
Sheaths, etheric/astral/egoic, 36
Solar plexus, effect on chakras, 48

Also by Ambika Wauters

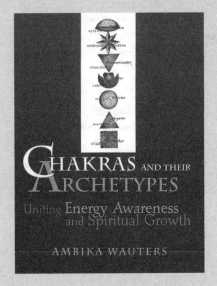

Chakras and Their Archetypes
Uniting Energy Awareness and Spiritual Growth

$16.95 PAPER
7 x 9 INCHES
176 PAGES
ISBN-13: 978-0-89594-891-5
ISBN-10: 0-89594-891-5

In CHAKRAS AND THEIR ARCHETYPES, Ambika Wauters relates archetypes to the chakras and guides us on a journey to understand where our energy is blocked and which attitudes or emotional issues are responsible. Using a variety of exercises, meditations, and affirmations, she helps us free ourselves from the negative archetypes, enabling us to rise to higher levels of awareness and empowerment—where we can transcend limitations, make healthy choices, release creativity, heal our pasts, and live with joy, vitality, and love.

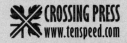

CROSSING PRESS
www.tenspeed.com